NutriScore

NutriScore

The Rate-Yourself Plan
for Better Nutrition

Ruth Fremes and Dr. Zak Sabry

Continuum • New York

1981
The Continuum Publishing Company
575 Lexington Avenue
New York, N.Y. 10022

Printed in the United States of America

Library of Congress Cataloging in Publication Data

Fremes, Ruth, 1930-
  NutriScore: the rate-yourself plan for better nutrition.

  Includes index.
  1. Nutrition   2. Food.   3. Diet.   I. Sabry, Zak,
1932-   II. Title.
TX353.F78   1981   641.1   81-9677
ISBN 0-8264-0056-6 (pbk.)   AACR2

Preface

NutriScore received such enthusiastic support from everyone—readers, media, students—that we felt the need to update and expand it. Many of you wrote to us, tracking us down at times through our publisher, and at other times, at our places of work. We enjoyed the compliments we received, but particularly appreciated the suggestions that you gave us to improve and expand future editions of NutriScore.

To you then, we dedicate this edition.

Contents

The
Rating
Game

Chapter 1
Nourishing Food Is Your Lifeline

Healthful eating and delicious food are synonymous. What we hope to accomplish by writing this book is to convince everyone of the truth of this statement. In our opinion it's shocking how the public is being cheated, and is cheating itself, of the rewards of good food. Instead of true orange flavor we get "orange taste." Instead of real juice we get a chemical drink. Instead of facts we get double-talk. We deserve better.

NutriScore is designed with you in mind. It is your map of the territory. Once you've familiarized yourself with the map and adapted it to your own eating habits, you can travel the supermarket highways with confidence. Now is not a moment too soon.

In underdeveloped countries, nutrition has been a life-and-death concern for many years. People don't have enough to eat. Their surroundings are unsanitary. Many people, particularly infants and children, succumb to infections and die. But who would think of malnutrition in the United States and Canada and other developed countries? It's happening.

For a long time when we thought of malnutrition we pictured starving Biafran or Vietnamese children; apathetic-looking, with skinny arms and legs and bloated stomachs. Little did we know that the prosperous executive with his double chin and huge girth might also be malnourished.

We are now realizing that a well-fed person is not necessarily a well-nourished person. Eating a lot and getting the nourishment we need are two different things.

We can only get the nourishment we need by eating a variety of foods that give us the fuel and the building blocks our bodies need. If we don't follow a proper diet, the consequences are serious, and we will pay for our mistakes sooner or later. Women who are malnourished before and during pregnancy are jeopardizing the health of their offspring. Their babies could be born with physical and/or mental handicaps or develop behavior and learning problems. A malnourished mother usually is not knowledgable enough to ensure that her

2

children are well nourished and the problem carries on from generation to generation.

It is estimated that 10 to 20 million people die every year from diseases directly or indirectly related to malnutrition. In addition to the nutritional deficiency diseases such as protein-calorie malnutrition, anemias, scurvy and rickets, there are obesity, coronary heart diseases, diabetes, cirrhosis of the liver, ulcers, kidney stones, and various types of cancer. In the United States and Canada poor eating habits contribute to the occurrence of coronary heart disease, North America's number one killer, which is responsible for 40 per cent of all deaths every year.

The cost of medical and dental care of diseases related to malnutrition is astronomical, well in excess of 30 billion dollars a year in the United States, and a billion and a half dollars a year in Canada. This is inexcusable, considering that much of the malnutrition in these countries is preventable.

A recent national survey in the United States found 95 per cent of children up to five years of age and women between the ages of 18 and 44 have below-standard iron intakes. There is also widespread shortage of calcium and vitamin A in the diets of women and children, particularly those on low incomes. In Canada there are an estimated 1½ million adults who are grossly obese; nearly 3 million adults with high blood cholesterol, which exposes them to the risk of heart attacks; 1½ million men, women, and children who lack adequate iron, resulting in reduced stamina, vitality, and productivity; and nearly 2 million children and teenagers who do not get enough calcium, thereby weakening bones in later life.

The responsibility for this state of affairs falls on many shoulders: Food companies who tamper with nourishing foods in an effort to present them attractively and thereby lower their nutritional value; doctors who emphasize medication and ignore the value of good eating; governments that are reluctant to show interest in the nutritional well-being of their citizens; and consumers who, helpless as they might be, do not make an effort to learn about nutrition and proper food preparation or to demand more nourishing foods in the marketplace, better medical service from their doctors, and sounder food regulation and nutrition service from their governments.

The majority of consumers, however, are at a disadvantage in the marketplace. Faced with an estimated 10 000 food items in the supermarket, they lack the technical knowledge to distinguish between those with high nutritional value and those that are junk. There is no easy system, and much of the information on nutrition in popular books and magazines only contributes to the confusion and leads to fad diets, many of which are dangerous. Some are written by misguided physicians, and the public is at a loss as to whom to believe. Several levels of government publish a wide variety of dull pamphlets, which, although reliable, seldom attract attention. The efforts of governments to promote nutrition knowledge lag far behind the food industry's efforts to promote their products.

The problem of difficult choices also exists in restaurants. It is estimated that North Americans eat one or two of every three meals away from home. It is increasingly common to eat breakfast at a coffee shop, lunch and snacks at the school or company cafeteria, and dinner from a fast-service or take-out chicken, hamburger, or pizza place. A glance at the alternatives offered at these establishments consistently shows that it is very difficult to order a nutritious meal. We are forced to order dishes that lack important vitamins and minerals.

As long as the food manufacturing and service companies ignore nutrition, consumers will have to take matters into their own hands. We will have to learn about nutrition to make intelligent decisions in the marketplace. Knowledge is the answer.

It is not true that our bodies automatically crave a specific food or nutrient they lack. We can tell when we are hungry and when we are thirsty, but when a fat man's stomach signals for more bread, it's because he's accustomed to large amounts. If the little boy's taste buds demand a rich dessert it's because he's learned to love sweets from the cradle on. Even when the worn-out young mother longs for a grilled cheese sandwich, her craving comes not from her body's need for fats and proteins and carbohydrates to replenish its energy, but more likely from some memory of childhood lunches or late-night snacks as a carefree teenager.

Other animals have better nutritional instincts. In repeated studies, nutrition researchers have offered rats two cups of food, identical in flavor and aroma but one more balanced nutritionally than the other. They observed that the rats chose the healthful food every time. Not only do rats sense which foods are best to eat, but when a cup of good food is replaced by a cup of nutritionally poor food, the rats go on a hunger strike. They would rather starve than switch. People, however, lack the rat's instinct to know when they're being offered poor nourishment, and worse, they often appear not to care.

Fortunately what we lack in nutritional instinct we make up for in intellect. People have become aware over the years that good food contributes to good health. After centuries of experimentation we now know a great deal about foods and their effect on the human body.

Naturally, the technological advances of the last century have speeded up the accumulation of nutritional knowledge. We now have complicated scientific equipment for experiments and analysis and computers to tabulate the results, so that we can examine our foods and ourselves thoroughly and accurately. Modern nutritionists know an enormous amount about what makes us healthy.

It's up to you to learn, too, not only the basic chemistry of nutrition, but the effects of that chemistry. This book gives you lots of information (some surprising and some shocking) about foods and your nutritional needs but, before you look at that, rate yourself with NutriScore in the next chapter.

REMEMBER

Don't be gulled; healthful eating and delicious food can mean the same thing.

We have become a nation of overfed and undernourished children, teens and adults.

In the United States and Canada, coronary heart disease, linked to poor eating habits, contributes to an estimated 40 per cent of all deaths.

Choosing is confusing! There are more than 12 000 food products sold today.

Don't rely on instinct! Rats instinctively select nourishing food, humans don't.

Let's learn—use NutriScore, rate your diet and choose with certainty.

Healthful eating is the reward: NutriScore is the way.

Chapter 2

The NutriScore Plan—
The Rate-Yourself Way to Better
Nutrition

Here is a scene that will sound familiar. Summer is here—and so, too, is a roll of fat around your midriff.

You swear off cereal, bread, and potatoes. You manage for a week and then you find yourself heading ever more frequently to the refrigerator for a snack or drink. You weigh yourself and find you've only lost a pound. You feel rotten, so you pull a baggy shirt over your bathing suit and head for . . . a submarine sandwich.

The really terrible part is that you may not have been eating too much bread or potato in the first place. Those extra calories could have come from food your body doesn't need very much, or can do without entirely.

Think of the unnecessary amount of fat that you may eat. If you use cream instead of milk with your breakfast cereal and coffee, or have fried eggs rather than soft-boiled or poached, or lunch on cream soup and a ham-and-cheese sandwich loaded with mayonnaise, you've had more fat than necessary. Cereal and bread are not the culprits if you gain weight on such a menu; and to cut them out completely deprives you of nutrients you need. But, you could do without cream and mayonnaise indefinitely and be all the better for it.

How can you tell if you're eating correctly? You could go to a nutritionist, recount in minute detail exactly what you eat every day and receive an analysis of your diet showing its strengths and weaknesses. This is not unlike a session with a psychoanalyst, because in both cases you tend to forget, or even suppress, important facts such as that second scoop of ice cream.

Or, you can rate your own diet using the NutriScore plan. Discover for yourself the strong points and the weak spots in your eating habits—*and* how to correct the balance.

NutriScore is the rating system we have designed for you to use. It gives you the most freedom and, therefore, the best assurance of success. We developed it by examining a large volume of data on what people eat and what foods provide which nutrients in our diets. We computerized where proteins, vitamins, minerals, and calories come from, and we organized these foods into eight groups. Then we assigned relative values to them and devised the NutriScore rating chart for you to use in scoring your diet. (Metric note: The "calories" we commonly refer to are, in fact, kilocalories.)

The NutriScore rating chart is on pages 11 to 25. As you read the following instructions, look it over. It is easy to use once you know the system.

Think of the NutriScore chart all the time. Part of the system involves keeping track of everything you eat for one week. Don't rely on memory. Write down what you eat and how much, and transfer this to the chart each day. Use pencil when you write on the chart. Then you can erase it and use it for other weeks.

INSTRUCTIONS

How to use the NutriScore chart. Foods have been broken down into eight areas designated as A through H. For one week, every time you eat anything, find the food in the appropriate area of the chart and fill in a square in the row next to it. If you can't find a food in the A through H chart area groupings, look in Appendix A where foods are listed alphabetically. Next to the alphabetical food listing you will find a reference to the area of the chart it corresponds to and to the item number in that area which it equals. (For example, next to the listing for Almonds in Appendix A it says A14. Fill in a square on the chart next to the entry for A14.) Appendix A also gives the caloric values of all the foods in the NutriScore chart.

Note honestly the size of servings. Remember to help yourself to seconds or thirds on the chart if that's what you did at the table! And if you have double helpings, fill in two squares. Also, don't forget to note half-servings. They add up and contribute to your rating. Don't cheat. After all, nobody knows or cares but you, so if you cheat, you're only cheating yourself.

Keep track in this way for seven consecutive days.

How to score yourself. At the beginning of each area, A through H, there is a number called the desirable rating. This number represents a balanced rating for one week. Notice that this figure varies for young and old, for pregnant and nursing women and for people trying to reduce.

After seven days count up the number of squares you have filled in for each food. Multiply the number of filled-in squares by the figure given in the column headed "Factor" and put the answer in the column headed "Rating". (The factor reflects the amount of certain nutrients in a given food.)

Finally, add the ratings down the column in each of the eight (A through H) areas *separately* and put each total in the space marked "Total Rating for One Week." Compare your total in each area to the number given as the desirable rating.

How to interpret your score to balance your diet nutritionally. For a balanced diet you need specific amounts of food from seven of the eight areas—A through G—each week. The foods in areas A through G provide a nutritional balance in proportion to the desirable rating values specified. The foods in area H supply little or no nourishment. They are mostly calories—in other words, they are "empty" foods and should be avoided.

Where your score in an area matches the desirable rating for that area, your nutritional supplies are adequate. All you need to do in that area is keep on the same course. Most people find that in most of the areas they are on target. They discover that their eating patterns are largely correct and that they are weak in one or two specific areas.

Where your score falls short of the desirable rating, increase your consumption of foods in that area. You can do this either by eating a number of the low-factor foods or by concentrating on two or three of the foods with high-factor values. Learning to eat just a few unfamiliar high-factor foods is a painless way to improve your health.

Where your score is higher than the desirable rating, don't worry unless you have an overweight problem. (And in that case, read on.)

Don't change good habits, only poor ones. If you prefer carrots raw as a salad or a snack, then a diet which overlooks them may be depriving you of an excellent eating pattern. Why change a perfectly healthful and long-standing habit? Continue crunching.

On the other hand, if you don't eat any carrots at all, either make sure you get enough of equivalent foods or try every carrot recipe in your favorite cookbook—and maybe a few others too—until you find one you like.

Notice that there are different desirable ratings in some areas for young and old and for pregnant and nursing women. The reasons for this are explained in Chapters 11 through 14. Notice too, that the

NutriScore system has been tailored to help those trying to lose weight.

How NutriScore can help you reduce wisely. The rating levels for people trying to lose weight are lower in some areas. If you aim for these lower scores you will not be getting fewer calories but your diet will still be balanced.

If you want to count your calorie intake as well, refer to Appendix A beginning on page 216. This alphabetical listing of foods and their nutrient contents can help you find the caloric values of foods in the NutriScore chart and of others which may not be listed in the eight areas.

It would be unwise to try to hurry weight loss by eating less and scoring lower than the recommended figure. Your diet must be balanced even when you are reducing.

Notice that certain foods are shaded on the chart. These foods are not allowed at all if you are trying to lose weight. As you will see, all the foods in area H are shaded. This whole group is low on nutrients and high in calories. Unless you are physically active and have no weight problem, plan to do without them.

If you take vitamin mineral pills, notice that there is a square for vitamin mineral supplements in Areas A, B, C and E of the chart. If you take a multiple vitamin capsule, be sure to fill in the squares in each area. For example, if a supplement contains both iron and vitamin A, fill in squares A21 and E9.

Everybody can win. The aim of the game is to make all your nutrition areas, areas of strength. Re-, re-, and re-rating is part of the system. If your initial score is too low or too high, don't quit. The only contest is with yourself. Note what you need to do to improve, whether you have been over-indulging or under-indulging. Rate yourself as often and as much as possible. Then re-rate yourself.

Use NutriScore seasonally, every three months, to make sure you haven't fallen into bad habits. It's easy to do. In summer, for instance, fresh fruit and vegetables are at their most appealing and are available at reasonable cost. You should have no difficulty meeting nutritional quotas with them. In winter, however, you may have to make a more conscious effort to eat enough of these foods each day.

Don't forget the family. Cooks like to feel that all their effort in the kitchen will keep the family not only full but full of health. Rate all members of the family and make sure they're being served what they need. Or, better still, let them rate themselves. Give everyone a different colored pencil and let them fill in the squares in their own special color.

The idea behind the NutriScore plan is that if you see for yourself what foods you lack for good health, you'll start to include these missing foods in your meals. And this goes for everyone, young or old. Nobody wants to feel lethargic and sluggish. Nutritious eating will give you and every member of the family the health and vitality that comes with a well-balanced and imaginative diet.

REMEMBER

Don't fall into bad eating habits—you may be misinterpreting where your excessive calories are coming from.

You can seek nutritional counsel from a specialist, but NutriScore will do if for you right here and now.

Carefully record your daily food intake for a week. Fill in a square on the chart whenever you eat—item by item, portion by portion.

Note the size of the servings you eat—they're important in NutriScoring yourself. Don't cheat. You'll only cheat yourself.

There are eight areas in which you have to rate your food intake—rate each separately and compare your score to the desirable rating.

If you want to lose weight, don't exceed the rating level recommended for dieters and eliminate the foods which are shaded on the chart.

Rate, re-rate, and re-rate. If your initial score is low, don't quit. Just check your NutriScore chart and do what it calls for in order to improve.

Don't change your good eating habits, only your poor ones.

Check yourself at least once every three months to make sure that you are maintaining your good effort.

Don't forget the rest of the family. Have everyone fill in the chart in different colors or get extra books and let them fill in their own. The family that eats healthily stays healthy.

AREA

A

DESIRABLE RATINGS FOR ONE WEEK

30 for children; 40 for teenagers; 30 for men; 40 for women; 45 for pregnant and nursing women; 25 for dieters, avoiding shaded foods

*Note that if items A-2, A-5, A-7, A-8, A-9, A-10, A-13, A-15, A-18, and A-19 are eaten as a sandwich, check bread in Area G of this Chart.

†Check also Item B-1 for the cheese on the cheeseburger

Food Item (Size of Serving)	Number of Servings Eaten in a Week	Total Servings	Factor	Rating
1 Baked beans or chili con carne or lentils or peas (½ cup or 125 mL cooked)	□□□□□□□□□□□□□□□□□□□□□□□□□□□□□□□□		2	
2 Beef or veal, any cut (3 oz. or 85 g cooked*)	□□□□□□□□□□□□□□□□□□□□□□□□□□□□□□		3	
3 Beef and vegetable stew (1 cup or 250 mL) or meat pot pie (8 oz. or 225 g)	□□□□□□□□□□□□□□□□□□□□□□□□□□□		3	
4 Cabbage rolls (2 medium)	□□□□□□□□□□□□□□□□□□□□□□□□		2	
5 Chicken or turkey or goose or duck, any cut (3 oz. or 85 g cooked*)	□□□□□□□□□□□□□□□□□□□□□□□□□□□□□□□		1	
6 Chop suey or chow mein (1 cup or 250 mL)	□□□□□□□□□□□□□□□□□□□□□□□□□		2	

Food Item (Size of Serving)	Number of Servings Eaten in a Week	Total Servings	Factor	Rating
7 Egg, any type (cooked* 1 medium)			1	
8 Fish and shellfish except salmon (B–6) or sardines (A–18) (3 oz. or 85 g cooked*) or fish stew (1 cup or 250 mL)			1	
9 Hamburger or cheeseburger*† (1 without bun)			4	
10 Lamb, any cut (3 oz. or 85 g cooked*)			1	
11 Lasagna with meat (1 cup or 250 mL)			3	
12 Liver, kidney or heart, any animal (2 oz. or 60 g)			5	
13 Luncheon meats, paté, or cold cuts; e.g. salami, tongue, bologna* (2 slices or 1 oz. or 30 g)			1	
14 Nuts, any type, raw or roasted (¼ cup or 50 mL)			1	
15 Peanut butter* (2 tbsp. or 25 mL)			1	

#	Food		Rating
16	Pizza with meat and cheese (1 small or 1 piece)	□□□□□□□□□□□□□□	1
17	Pork, back bacon or ham, any cut (3 oz. or 85 g cooked*)	□□□□□□□□□□□□□□	2
18	Sardines* (3 oz. or 85 g)	□□□□□□□□□□□□□□	3
19	Sausages* (3 medium) including weiners* (1 medium)	□□□□□□□□□□□□□□	1
20	Spaghetti with meat sauce or macaroni and beef (1 cup or 250 mL)	□□□□□□□□□□□□□□	2
21	Vitamin/mineral supplement with iron (1 pill or capsule)	□□□□□□□□□□□□□□	1

Total Rating for One Week

B

DESIRABLE RATINGS FOR ONE WEEK

30 for children; 55 for teenagers; 40 for men; 40 for women; 70 for pregnant and nursing women; 30 for dieters.

Food Item (Size of Serving)	Number of Servings Eaten in a Week	Total Servings	Factor	Rating
1 Cheese, Cheddar, Swiss, process Canadian or American (1 oz. or 30 g)			2	
2 Cheese, cottage (½ cup or 125 mL)			1	
3 Macaroni and cheese (1 cup or 250 mL)			3	
4 Milk of any animal, whole, 2%, skim, buttermilk or chocolate (1 cup or 250 mL)			3	
5 Puddings, made with milk (½ cup or 125 mL)			1	
6 Salmon, canned with soft bones (3 oz. or 85 g)			2	

Food Item	Number of Servings Eaten in a Week	Total Servings	Factor	Rating
7 Soups made with milk (6 fl. oz. or 175 mL)	☐☐☐☐☐☐☐☐☐☐☐☐☐☐ ☐☐☐☐☐☐☐		1	
8 Yogurt any style (6 oz. or 175 mL)	☐☐☐☐☐☐☐☐☐☐☐☐☐☐ ☐☐☐☐☐☐☐		2	
9 Vitamin/mineral supplement with calcium (1 pill or capsule)	☐☐☐☐☐☐☐☐☐☐☐☐☐☐ ☐☐☐☐☐☐☐		1	

Total Rating for One Week

AREA

C

DESIRABLE RATING FOR ONE WEEK

7 for children, teenagers, men, women, pregnant and nursing women, and dieters.

Food Item (Size of Serving)	Number of Servings Eaten in a Week	Total Servings	Factor	Rating
1 Apple juice, vitaminized, vitamin C added (4 fl. oz. or 125 mL)	☐☐☐☐☐☐☐☐☐☐☐☐☐☐ ☐☐☐☐☐☐☐		1	
2 Avocado (1 medium)	☐☐☐☐☐☐☐☐☐☐☐☐☐☐ ☐☐☐☐☐☐☐		1	

		Rating
3	Berries, e.g. blueberries, raspberries, strawberries (¾ cup or 175 mL)	1
4	Cabbage, raw or cooked (½ cup or 125 mL)	1
5	Cantaloupe (¼ of medium sized)	1
6	Cauliflower (¾ cup or 175 mL cooked)	1
7	Grapefruit, fresh, canned or juice (½ medium size or ½ cup or 125 mL)	1
8	Orange, fresh, canned or juice (1 medium or ½ cup or 125 mL)	1
9	Pepper (1 medium)	1
10	Tangerine, fresh, canned or juice (1 medium or ½ cup or 125 mL)	1
11	Tomato, fresh, canned or juice (1 medium or ¾ cup or 175 mL)	1
12	Vitamin/mineral supplement with vitamin C or ascorbic acid (1 pill or capsule)	1

Total Rating for One Week

AREA

D

DESIRABLE RATING FOR ONE WEEK

7 for children, teenagers, men, women, pregnant and nursing women, and dieters.

Food Item (Size of Serving)	Number of Servings Eaten in a Week	Total Servings	Factor	Rating
1 Apple (1 medium) or applesauce (½ cup or 125 mL)	□□□□□□□□□□□□□□		1	
2 Banana (1 medium)	□□□□□□□□□□□□□□		1	
3 Dried fruits, e.g. raisins, dates, figs, prunes (1 oz. or 30 g)	□□□□□□□□□□□□□□		1	
4 Grapes, fresh or juice (½ cup or 125 mL)	□□□□□□□□□□□□□□		1	
5 Other fruits such as apricots, peaches pears, etc., or fruit cocktail (1 medium or ½ cup or 125 mL)	□□□□□□□□□□□□□□		1	

Total Rating for One Week

AREA

E

DESIRABLE RATING FOR ONE WEEK

14 for children, teenagers, men, women, pregnant and nursing women, and dieters.

Food Item (Size of Serving)	Number of Servings Eaten in a Week	Total Servings	Factor	Rating
1 Asparagus (½ cup or 125 mL cooked)	☐☐☐☐☐☐☐☐☐☐☐☐☐☐		2	
2 Broccoli (½ cup or 125 mL cooked)	☐☐☐☐☐☐☐☐☐☐☐☐☐☐		2	
3 Brussels sprouts (½ cup or 125 mL cooked)	☐☐☐☐☐☐☐☐☐☐☐☐☐☐		2	
4 Celery (½ cup or 125 mL)	☐☐☐☐☐☐☐☐☐☐☐☐☐☐		1	
5 Cucumber (4 slices)	☐☐☐☐☐☐☐☐☐☐☐☐☐☐		1	
6 Green leafy vegetables (½ cup or 125 mL cooked)	☐☐☐☐☐☐☐☐☐☐☐☐☐☐		2	
7 Lettuce, raw (2 leaves or ½ cup or 125 mL)	☐☐☐☐☐☐☐☐☐☐☐☐☐☐		2	

		Factor
8 Parsley (½ cup or 125 mL)	□□□□□□□□□□□□□□ □□	2
9 Vitamin/mineral supplement with vitamin A and folic acid (1 pill or capsule)	□□□□□□□□□□□□□□ □□	1

Total Rating for One Week

AREA

F

DESIRABLE RATING FOR ONE WEEK

10 for children, teenagers, men, women, pregnant and nursing women, and dieters.

Food Item (Size of Serving)	Number of Servings Eaten in a Week	Total Servings	Factor	Rating
1 Beans, green or yellow, or bean-sprouts (½ cup or 125 mL cooked)	□□□□□□□□□□□□□□□□□□□□□□		2	
2 Carrots, raw (1 medium), cooked (½ cup or 125 mL)	□□□□□□□□□□□□□□□□□		2	
3 Kale (½ cup or 125 mL cooked)	□□□□□□□□□□□□□□		2	

(Area F Cont'd.)

Food Item (Size of Serving)	Number of Servings Eaten in a Week	Total Servings	Factor	Rating
4 Peas or mixed vegetables (½ cup or 125 mL cooked)			1	
5 Potatoes, baked or boiled (1 medium) or mashed (½ cup or 125 mL) or scalloped or hash browned (¼ cup or 50 mL)			1	
6 Sweet potatoes or winter squash, such as Hubbard, or Acorn squash (½ cup or 125 mL)			2	
7 Turnip or summer squash, such as zucchini or butternut squash (½ cup or 125 mL)			1	
8 Other vegetables or salad (½ cup or 125 mL)			1	

Total Rating for One Week

AREA

G

DESIRABLE RATINGS FOR ONE WEEK

20 for children; 20 for teenagers; 20 for men; 20 for women; 25 for pregnant and nursing women; 10 for dieters.

Food Item (Size of Serving)	Number of Servings Eaten in a Week	Total Servings	Factor	Rating
1 Bread, white enriched or rye (1 slice)	□□□□□□□□□□□□□□□□□□□□□□		1	
2 Bread, whole grain, such as whole wheat (1 slice)	□□□□□□□□□□□□		2	
3 Cereal, enriched such as farina (¾ cup or 175 mL cooked)			1	
4 Cereal, enriched, ready-to-eat, unsweetened (1 oz. or 30 g or 1 cup or 250 mL)	□□□□□□□□□□□□□□□□□□□□□□		1	
5 Cereal, whole grain such as oatmeal (¾ cup or 175 mL cooked)	□□□□□□□□□□□□		2	
6 Cereal, whole grain, ready-to-eat, such as shredded wheat (1 oz. or 30 g)	□□□□□□□□□□□□		2	
7 Crackers, plain or fancy made with white flour (4 crackers)	□□□□□□□□□□□□□□□□		1	

Food Item (Size of Serving)	Number of Servings Eaten in a Week	Total Servings	Factor	Rating
8 Crackers, whole grain such as rye, Graham, wheat (4 crackers)	□□□□□□□□□□ □□□□□□□□□□		2	
9 Macaroni, noodles or spaghetti, plain or with tomato sauce (½ cup or 125 mL)	□□□□□□□□□□ □□□□□□□□□□		1	
10 Muffin or bun, made with white flour (a medium)	□□□□□□□□□□ □□□□□□□□□□		1	
11 Muffin or bun, made with bran or whole grain flour (1 medium)	□□□□□□□□□□ □□□□□□□□□□		2	
12 Pancake or waffles, plain (6″ or 15 cm diameter) or tea biscuits (2)	□□□□□□□□□□ □□□□□□□□□□		1	
13 Rice, parboiled, converted or brown (½ cup or 125 mL cooked)	□□□□□□□□□□ □□□□□□□□□□		2	
14 Rice, regular or instant (½ cup or 125 mL)	□□□□□□□□□□ □□□□□□□□□□		1	
15 Wheat bran or wheat germ (3 tbsp. or 50 mL)	□□□□□□□□□□ □□□□□□□□□□		2	

Total Rating for One Week

AREA

H

DESIRABLE RATINGS FOR ONE WEEK

Should not exceed 25 for children; teenagers; men; women; and pregnant and nursing women. Should be avoided by dieters.

Food Item (Size of Serving)	Number of Servings Eaten in a Week	Total Servings	Factor	Rating
1 Alcoholic beverages; beer (12 fl. oz. or 341 mL), wine 5 fl. oz. or 150 mL), or liquor (1¼ fl. oz. or 40 mL)			1	
2 Apple turnover (1 medium)			3	
3 Bacon, side (3 slices)			1	
4 Butter or margarine (1 tsp. or 5 mL) or cream or mayonnaise (1 tbsp. or 15 mL) or gravy (2 tbsp. or 25 mL)				
5 Cake with icing (2½" or 6 cm square) or brownies or squares (2 pieces)			2	
6 Cereal, sugar coated or pre-sweetened (1 oz. or 30 g)			1	
7 Chocolate bar, candy or fudge (1½ oz. or 42 g)			2	

Food Item (Size of Serving)	Number of Servings Eaten in a Week	Total Servings	Factor	Rating
8 Coffee or tea with cream and/or sugar (2 cups or 500 mL)	□□□□□□□□□□□□□□□□□□□□		1	
9 Cream cheese such as Philadelphia, Camembert or Roquefort (1 oz. or 30 g)	□□□□□□□□□□□□□□□□□□□□		1	
10 Donut, Danish pastry or Chelsea bun (1 medium) or cookies (2)	□□□□□□□□□□□□□□□□□□□□		1	
11 Egg roll (1 medium)	□□□□□□□□□□□□□□□□□□□□		2	
12 French fried potatoes or onion rings (10 pieces)	□□□□□□□□□□□□□□□□□□□□		2	
13 Fruit drinks with or without added vitamin C (1 cup or 250 mL)	□□□□□□□□□□□□□□□□□□□□		1	
14 Gelatin desserts, prepared with water (¾ cup or 175 mL)	□□□□□□□□□□□□□□□□□□□□		1	
15 Honey or jams and jellies (2 tbsp or 25 mL) or molasses (1 tbsp. or 15 mL) or sugar or syrups (2 tbsp. or 25 mL)	□□□□□□□□□□□□□□□□□□□□		1	
16 Ice cream or sherbet, any flavor (¾ cup or 175 mL)	□□□□□□□□□□□□□□□□□□□□		2	

17	Milk shakes, hot chocolate, or sundaes, any flavor (1 cup or 250 mL)	☐☐☐☐☐☐☐☐☐☐☐☐☐☐	2
18	Pancake or waffle with butter and syrup (6" or 15 cm square)	☐☐☐☐☐☐☐☐☐☐☐☐☐☐	3
19	Pie, any flavor (⅙ of 9" or 22 cm piece)	☐☐☐☐☐☐☐☐☐☐☐☐☐☐	4
20	Popcorn, salted and buttered (2 cups or 500 mL)	☐☐☐☐☐☐☐☐☐☐☐☐☐☐	1
21	Potato chips, corn chips and other fried snacks (1 cup or 250 mL)	☐☐☐☐☐☐☐☐☐☐☐☐☐☐	2
22	Soft drinks, carbonated or non-carbonated, any flavor, regular (non-diet) (10 fl. oz. or 300 mL)	☐☐☐☐☐☐☐☐☐☐☐☐☐☐	1

Total Rating for One Week

Dieting
and the
Calorie-Makers

Chapter 3

Dieting, or Balancing the Calorie-Makers with the Calorie-Spenders

NutriScore gives you an excellent opportunity to eat well and lose weight; simply reach and do not exceed the rating level specified in each area for dieters. At the same time step up your exercise program gradually and watch your weight drop. Once you have reached your goal, adjust your score and keep up your exercise. In the long run, it is the best diet program there is. It allows you to lose weight safely and improve your eating habits for good.

Speaking of diets. A friend in the publishing business tells us that the word "diet" on a magazine cover sells more copies than the word "sex," probably because one in every three teenagers and adults is estimated to be "on a diet." (What this indicates about sex we won't say, although we will mention that there is no aphrodisiac like the glow of good health). Unfortunately, all this dieting hasn't done adults in North America much good.

Why have our diets failed? If three-quarters of us have dieted, yet half of us are still overweight, something, if you'll excuse the pun, is grossly wrong. We think the difficulty is that most diets do not conform to our eating habits. By the time we become adults we have formed definite habits, attitudes, preferences and prejudices against certain foods. Any diet that is going to succeed, any diet you are going to persevere with, must take these habits into account.

Don't just pick up any diet. You shouldn't get it on a friend's recommendation or from a magazine or book, the way you buy a painkiller or cough medicine off the shelf. You should even be wary of doctors who hand out diet sheets the way they give a routine prescription. How many of them would question you closely enough to find out that you're fat because you can't stand lettuce, so you eat a second helping of meat while the rest of the family attacks the salad bowl? That's the sort of thing doctors should know before prescribing a diet.

A diet is a way of life. After all, what is the use of following your friend's recommendation of spinach and cottage cheese, or your doctor's recipe for boiled fish five times a week, if you resolve never to touch spinach or cottage cheese or fish again once those twenty pounds are gone? The twenty pounds will soon be back and you won't be able to face another diet. A diet should contain the foods you should eat for good health every day of your life in slightly reduced amounts; foods you can conveniently prepare or purchase, foods you can afford and, most of all, foods you can eat with pleasure.

If you have or suspect medical problems, don't diet without consulting your doctor. If you have diabetes or any other metabolic disease, only your doctor is qualified to judge how a change in diet will affect your health. If your nausea and indigestion come from gall bladder trouble, don't go on your neighbor's gall bladder diet. Go to your physician. Your gall bladder trouble might turn out to be ulcers, a spastic colon, or even a pregnancy, and your diet should be different in every case. NEVER DIAGNOSE AND TREAT DISEASES. The risk is too great. Only a physician should treat illness.

If you have a disease that requires specific foods to be eliminated from your diet, ask your doctor to refer you to a registered dietitian. You need someone who is knowledgable about foods and nutrition with whom you can discuss your problem. Dietary services are often not available at physicians' clinics but you could be referred to a special dietary clinic at the nearest hospital. Your registered dietitian knows the nutritional value of each food you buy and how it is affected by cooking and processing. She (not many men have entered this specialty) knows your requirements for calories, protein, vitamins, and minerals. She can help you substitute other foods for those you must avoid without aggravating your diabetes or any other illness you may have, and without missing an important vitamin or mineral, which could result in malnutrition.

If you merely need to lose weight, eat less and do more. Farmers who want fat hogs, geese and steers keep them penned up and eating. Trainers of race horses and managers of boxers rely on a combination of rationing and exercise to keep their charges trim. To get slim and stay trim, the simple secret is: eat less and do more, but always in moderation. You shouldn't cut your eating to a *lot* less, because too sharp a reduction in food intake is hard on the body and can't be maintained over any length of time. And don't suddenly do a *lot* more, because a sudden increase in physical effort can be too great a strain. You need to exercise more than usual to burn up more of the fat you already have plus what you continue to take in. In other words, our bodies must spend more calories than they receive. The calorie-spending (exercise) must outweigh the calorie-making (eating).

To maintain a desirable weight after you have reached it, add a few calories so that the income is no longer less than the expenditure, but exactly the same. When the calorie-makers balance the calorie-spenders and when both are in correct proportions, you should be in top shape.

The calorie-makers are the fats, carbohydrates and proteins in the foods you eat and the drinks you drink. The calorie-spenders are your basal metabolic needs and physical activity. The basal metabolic needs constitute the energy your body needs to exist without any activity, almost in a motionless state. It is a fairly constant amount from day to day, although it decreases as you grow older and increases as you grow bigger. Calories spent in physical activity may vary from day to day depending on what you do. The more you walk, run, swim, ski, play and generally use your muscles, the more calories you spend.

Reduce, but don't unbalance, the calorie-makers. A balanced diet should consist of about 30 percent of calories from fat, 60 percent from carbohydrates and 10 percent from protein. Recent statistics on food consumption show that the overall diet in North America is made up of about 45 percent of calories from fat, approximately 40 percent from carbohydrates and nearly 15 percent from protein. We are eating much too much fat and not enough carbohydrates. The balance among the three sources of calories should be maintained regardless of the total calories in the diet. To lose weight, you must reduce the number of calories consumed, not merely the proportions of fats, carbohydrates, and proteins.

How to lose weight by spending calories. What do you have to do to lose that extra poundage? Well, to lose an average of one pound a week (which is safe to attempt without medical attention), the weekly deficit must be 3500 calories, or 500 calories per day. For an adult normally living on 2000 calories, a deficit of 500 calories could be achieved by lowering the intake by 300 calories and increasing activity by 200 calories. This shouldn't be hard to do, for 300 out of 2000 calories is a very small sacrifice. Think of what you can do by cutting down on rich desserts (a piece of pastry or cake could mean 250 calories) or sugar in coffee or tea (sweetening six cups daily with sugar could mean 150 calories) or butter on your toast (50 calories for two pieces of toast). Walking three miles or swimming for 20 minutes would burn up the other 200 calories.

The following table gives the number of calories you would burn in various physical activities. Choose your sport and lose weight.

Caloric Expenditure for Various Sports
Average for Young Adults

Canoeing (4 mph or 6.4 km/h)	420 calories per hour
Horseback riding (trot)	480 calories per hour
Playing tennis	210 calories per 30 minutes
Swimming	160 calories per 20 minutes
Cross country skiing (level ground)	600 calories per hour
Cross country skiing (uphill)	190 calories per 10 minutes
Cross country running	121 calories per 10 minutes
Bicycling	180 calories per 30 minutes
Jogging	100 calories per 10 minutes
Brisk walking	150 calories per 30 minutes
Playing football	270 calories per 30 minutes
Dancing	120 calories per 15 minutes

Physical activity makes it easier to eat less and to stay slim. Experiments on both animals and men have proved the truth of this statement. For example, Dr. Jean Mayer, who studied the problem of obesity for many years, examined 300 workers ranging from secretary-clerks and tailors to blacksmiths and coalmen. These manual workers' food intake was self-regulated since they lived away from their families and ate in a remarkably uniform pattern. The analysis of the results accounted for weights, heights, caloric intakes, physical activity as well as economic differences, cultural differences, and ethnic factors. The study showed that men "with regular moderate activity ate somewhat less and *were considerably thinner* than the inactive ones."

Our bodies are designed and constructed for activity. Our ancestors would not have survived the harsh conditions of primitive life had their bodies not been in top physical shape. We must remember that we still need to run for our lives!

Exercise is a pleasure and a duty. There are two kinds of exercise: the first is our normal daily activities and the second is what we do specifically to keep fit. Don't underestimate everyday exercise. We depend on simple movement to keep our muscles toned, and anyone who has ever been immobilized by illness for a week or so has felt the terrible flaccidity of unexercised muscles. Astronauts, men and women in peak physical condition, find themselves wobbly on return to earth because in the weightlessness of space their muscles no longer have the pull of gravity to work against and rapidly lose their tone. The benefits of exercise cannot be stored; exercise has to be repeated regularly. Like Alice in Wonderland, we have to keep running in order to stay in the same place.

Exercising to keep fit, on the other hand, moves us ahead. An adult walking a mile every day uses up about 75 calories whether it takes him 15 or 30 minutes. But jogging that mile in 9 minutes every day would give you the added advantages of toning muscles, improving blood circulation, increasing stamina, and reducing fatigue.

It's legal to get hooked on exercise and it's one habit that's healthy to form. As we've said, we're all addicted to the extent that we have to exercise regularly in order to continue to function. To lose weight and improve fitness, we must increase the amount and exertion of the exercise and still do it regularly. The condition of the muscles deteriorates and the body's ability to burn excess fat lags when we let the habit slide.

Put your effort into the exercise, not into getting ready to exercise. Waiting until your name comes up on the list at the country club is an excuse, not an exercise. You don't need to join an expensive health spa, either. Without spending a cent you can walk all the way to work, or at least part way, or you can find a like-minded friend and plan a half-hour jaunt at lunch break. Increase your pace gradually, and keep it up every day, not excluding weekends, when you can introduce your family and friends to the great out-of-doors. The exercise doesn't have to be the same every day. You can walk Monday and Wednesday, swim Tuesday and Thursday and ski all weekend, as long as the amount of exercise you receive remains constant. A day of ironing, or a day of entertaining a tedious business associate cannot replace an all-day hike. So, have fun with a clear conscience; it's good for your health.

The grain-of-salt diets. We all know that calories *do* count and that the way to reduce is to cut down on caloric intake while stepping up caloric output. Yet every so often some charm school instructor, food faddist, self-styled nutritionist or medical doctor who has forgotten most of what he once knew pops up with a "new, revolutionary diet." We call these grain-of-salt diets because that's how you should take them.

The trouble with fad diets is that they are unbalanced. Our bodies require specific amounts of the many different nutrients (the rest of this section and the next section of the book are devoted to discussion of these nutrients and where they are found). If these nutrients are not eaten in the right amounts, the body is in trouble, and eventually so are we. Instead of taking the sensible course of cutting back a little bit, these diets advocate extremes. There are low-carbohydrate diets; low-carbohydrate but high-fat diets; low carbohydrate, high-protein diets; and low-protein, high-carbohydrate diets. Each proponent assures us that his is the only diet worth following.

Dr. Stillman's Quick Weight Loss Diet is low in carbohydrate but high in protein. His Inches-Off Diet reverses this theory to prescribe a lot of carbohydrates but a minimum of proteins.

The Scarsdale Diet is very similar to Stillman's Quick Weight Loss Diet. It prescribes a great deal of protein but is nutritionally unbalanced. It is low in calcium and vitamin A because of an almost total absence of dairy products. Its success is more probably due to its paternalistic tone than to any nutritional or dieting sense. It is rigid, but recognizes its rigidity and allows the dieter relief in 14-day cycles. It sets limits on the foods but not the amounts. This on-again off-again dieting merry-go-round sets everyone running around in circles. It is healthier and safer to keep on a balanced diet. Learn to control the amounts you eat and do it forever.

Dr. Atkins' Diet concentrates on reduction of carbohydrates in the diet, and allows relatively higher intakes of fat. The American Medical Association Council on Foods and Nutrition concluded that Dr. Atkins' low-carbohydrate, high-fat diet is "for the most part without scientific merit and not only that, it is also potentially dangerous." (Unfortunately the A.M.A. Council does not possess Dr. Atkins' personal charisma, nor does it have the advantage of an aggressive public relations staff to promote its message.)

Severely reducing carbohydrates, as Dr. Atkins recommends, can seriously lower your blood sugar, making you hypoglycemic. You are cutting off a vital source of energy for the brain and muscles. It's no wonder that many of Dr. Atkins' diet followers feel tired and cranky. In addition, the high fat intake he advises help build up cholesterol and other fat in the blood, and increases the risk of heart disease. The extra vitamin pills recommended with the diet do not help the situation. The problem with the diet is that the sources of energy are not balanced. The body cannot live on fat alone; it needs carbohyrates as well.

What's more, remember Dr. Atkins' warning about body odors: as your blood sugar level drops, fat is utilized to provide energy to the body. But the fat is not completely broken down and chemicals known as ketone bodies are formed. They smell terrible and since they are emitted through the lungs you can count on being less than kissing fresh.

The low carbohydrate, high-fat diet isn't good for anyone. For pregnant women and people with heart disease it's a menace.

Fasting is another fad. Often the proponents fast not only to lose weight but to "cleanse their bodies." Whatever the reason, fasting can be dangerous. What actually happens when we fast is that the body literally "eats itself." Tissues are broken down and their contents recycled with part being burned for energy. Here, we are not burning fat, we are burning tissues, fat, protein, the works. Vitamins and minerals are lost from the body and their supply not replenished. You get the fatigue symptoms associated with hypoglycemia without the smelly ketosis. You are seriously endangering your health the longer you carry it on. Occasionally you hear of a doctor hospitalizing an obese patient and starving him to thinness. But this is very tricky business even under doctor's supervision, let alone doing it on your own.

Pritikin's Maximum Weight Loss Diet was described as "superior by far to any fast." In might be better than nothing but it should be avoided. In both the 600 and 1000 calorie versions, the diet falls short of many nutrients, including protein. The demand it places for excessive amounts of vegetables makes it difficult to follow for long periods of time.

Yet another diet by Pritikin, the Longevity Diet, makes sense. With slightly more calories, 1200-1500 a day, it is adequate in protein, low in fat, saturated fat and cholesterol, low in sodium, and high in fiber. Dieters can lose weight slowly and safely on such a diet. In fact, Pritikin's Longevity goes beyond dieting to require followers to give up smoking and to exercise regularly. In all, the program encourages healthful living habits.

There are a hundred and one other fad diets. There is the *Drinking Man's Diet*, which has got to be a joke because drinking alcohol while restricting foods is a harmful way to treat your body. Then there is the *Grapefruit Diet*, which gives you the benefit of a lot of vitamin C, but this does *not* melt away the fat when eaten before (or after, or in the middle of) a meal.

The diets we recommend are those that qualify as "low calorie" diets. They help you cut down on calories while keeping your diets balanced. Examples of these diets are: Pritikin's Longevity Diet (by Nathan Pritikin and Patrick McGrady, published by Grosset and Dunlap, New York, 1979), The Prudent Diet (by Iva Bennett and Martha Simon, published by David White, New York, 1973), The New York Health Department Diet (in a pamphlet entitled "Eat to Lose Weight," published by the Bureau of Nutrition, Department of Health, City of New York, 93 Worth Street, New York, N.Y. 10013).

Considering the way we eat in North America, it pays to endorse the Dietary Guidelines proposed by the United States Department of Agriculture and the Department of Health and Human Services to: "eat a variety of foods; maintain ideal weight; avoid too much fat, saturated fat and cholesterol; eat food with adequate starch and fiber; avoid too much sugar; avoid too much sodium; and if you drink alcohol, do so in moderation." There are a number of booklets produced by these government departments outlining menus to help follow these guidelines. Pritikin's Longevity Diet and the Prudent Diet are consistent with these guidelines.

Designing your own NutriScore Diet should work best of all. Choose the foods you like from each area. Make sure your nutritional score is at the level specified in each area for those trying to lose weight, no more and no less. Then eliminate completely the foods which are shaded and cut down the size of serving of each food you do eat by one-quarter the amount, *no more.* Stay at this level and exercise regularly and you'll drop pounds and feel great.

Club your weight down. Most reducers look for support from other people and these days there is a proliferation of "clubs" looking for overweight people to join. As with diets, some clubs are sound and helpful and some are ineffective, money-wasting and potentially harmful.

The useful weight loss clubs are those based on group discussion and sound nutrition and exercise programs. They include Weight Watchers, Diet Workshop, and Take Off Pounds Sensibly (TOPS). These clubs operate on a very simple principle: dieting and exercising are lonely activities. In these clubs, members join social support as they meet regularly to discuss their problems and share their achievements. In addition to social support Weight Watchers provides sound medical and nutritional advice.

We do not, however, support clubs which sell foods for dieters, such as the TV-dinner-type products sold under the Weight Watchers or similar labels. In the first place, this kind of convenience food is subjected to extensive processing and handling that may lower its content of vitamins and minerals. Also, it is restrictive and, if you rely heavily on these foods, you could be missing a lot of nutrients you get from a varied diet. The only advantage these foods offer, besides convenience, is a statement on the label of the number of calories they contain. We think most foods sold in our supermarkets should carry this information on their label, and in fact, restaurants should state it on their menus.

Joining these clubs costs money and, if you can't afford it, you might get a group together, sponsor one person to find out how the club works, then form a similar club of your own. On occasion, it's worth paying a membership fee, and it may not cost as much as you think. An elderly lady we know was becoming more and more housebound, partly because of rheumatoid arthritis and partly because of a retired and ailing husband. She knew that she was eating too much but hadn't the heart to diet until the doctor decided that her weight was aggravating her arthritis. A diet club located in a nearby church offered a Senior Citizen's membership for a dollar, and thanks to it she got out of the house, met some new people, heard the latest about nutrition, was encouraged to stay with her diet, and at last report had lost seventeen pounds. She says she felt foolish and frivolous dieting alone at her age, but when she talked about it within the group, her diet became important and worthwhile. She doesn't adhere exactly to the diet because her husband has special dietary requirements and she doesn't want to cook two separate meals, but she has grasped the nutritional principles and follows them. She hasn't been so slim since her forties and never intends to gain weight again.

Exercise clubs are useful if you use them, but you don't need them. Walking, jogging, swimming, snowshoeing and cross country skiing can all be done without joining anything. Ask a friend to join *you*, and that's all the club you need. However, if you do put out money to join an exercise club, go there as often as possible and use all the equipment. Exercise clubs and spas make money because such a small percentage of their clients use the facilities. A friend of ours joined a $300-a-year health club and estimates that it cost him $50 per hour to exercise. If he could get there four or five times a week the cost would be reduced to $1.50 per session.

The clubs or groups to distrust are the ones that promise you painless weight loss. They usually start their advertisement or sales talk by pointing out that they are different from the other clubs. They have a magic method that uses equipment or devices exclusively theirs. One such outfit advertises:

> *"We give you a good plan that you can live with. You just relax and let our special equipment to go to work on you . . . for you . . . gently, and you never disrobe . . . the weight comes off.*
> *"Results guaranteed on recommended programs. No crash dieting. No strenuous exercise."*

Many of these outfits offer you a free courtesy visit or a block of several visits at a special introductory price. Their hope, and they often succeed, is that you will succumb to the heavy, persuasive sales talk and sign up for the year or longer.

Forget those weight-reducing devices at exorbitant prices. Whatever they are called, whatever magazine they're in, however they claim to work, they're no good. Many are wraps or garments worn over certain parts of the body. Some heat up and others vibrate. Some are supposed to work on the sauna principle, that is, you lose water and therefore weight ... for a few hours. Some speak of magic. We say baloney. Anyone who claims you can lose weight without diet and exercise is a fraud. The only device that can accomplish your weight loss is a thing called YOU, and as for effortless exercise, it's a contradiction in terms, physically impossible and intellectually illogical. To expect you to believe it is an insult to your judgment and intelligence.

The drugged dieter is in trouble. The use of drugs is the most reprehensible method of treating obesity. It started in the early 1940s with the discovery that amphetamine, a brain stimulant, suppresses appetite. Drug houses promoted amphetamines as a treatment for obesity. By the 1960s the market was flooded with amphetamine and its derivatives. Some physicians found a lucrative new specialty: by 1968, the Food and Drug Administration estimated that 5000 to 7000 physicians in the United States were practicing as "fat doctors." These fat doctors got the whole thing down to a fine art. With the help of drug companies, they dispensed "rainbow" pills, pills of different colors meant to be taken in a certain sequence. They included amphetamines to suppress appetite, barbiturates to counter the nervousness caused by amphetamines, thyroxine and other hormones to increase the basal metabolic rate, diuretics to flush water from the body, and laxatives to move food out of the intestines before it was absorbed. Sometimes the collection of pills included digitalis, a heart muscle stimulant. Many of these drugs, such as amphetamine, thyroxine, and digitalis, tax the heart severely. Furthermore, the diuretics such as thiazide increase the loss of potassium and make the heart dangerously sensitive to digitalis.

There is a distinct danger is prescribing amphetamine and there is no evidence of its value in the treatment of obesity. This is why amphetamines are no longer allowed for use to suppress appetite. Yet, it was not long ago that they were readily prescribed. The number of prescriptions rose through the 1960s; in 1967, eight billion doses of amphetamines were produced in the United States. In that same year, the number of new prescriptions of amphetamines in the United

States was about 15 million plus 31 million refills. By 1971, the number of new prescriptions was over 26 million.

Reports of sudden and unexpected deaths among consumers of amphetamines began to accumulate in the 1960s in impressive numbers. From Oregon State University came the case of a co-ed who fought obesity with "rainbow" pills until she got her weight down to where she had always wanted it. A year later and for no apparent reason she dropped dead in her dormitory. The suspected cause: the rainbow pills. Dr. Russell Henry, Oregon State Medical Investigator at the time, stated that he knew of possibly seven other women who had died the same way.

A report from Illinois about the same time linked the sudden and unexpected death of fourteen young people to the "diet" pill. More reports of similar deaths started filing in. In 1968 a U.S. Senate subcommittee opened hearings into the obesity business. Five years later, the Food and Drug Administration decided to revise the labelling of amphetamines "to more thoroughly describe the limitations of their use." By the mid-seventies, health authorities in the United States and Canada limited the use of amphetamines to specific conditions that did *not* include diet control.

The fact remains that there are many people who are dissatisfied with themselves, and will risk their health for a promise of a "better," slimmer figure. This alone shows us that there is much to be learned about overweight and its control, both medically and psychologically. Not only must dieters take their problem seriously but, in our opinion, the medical profession must offer support, comfort and advice to patients beginning the long, slow trek towards their ideal weight.

Losing weight is a slow business. You don't put on weight quickly and you shouldn't take it off too quickly either. Be satisfied to cut your calories by only a quarter of your normal daily needs. If you make it any more severe, you will be getting less than the required amount of protein, vitamins and minerals. You want to go from thick to thin not from thick to sick.

The same applies to exercise. Too much sudden exercise may tax the body's capabilities and lead to exhaustion. Start at a level you can take with mild effort and built up gradually to greater feats.

There are lots of shady characters in the diet business ready to promise a new you without any effort. Beware of them. What do you want with a new you, anyway? What you want is the *old* in prime condition. All it costs is time and effort. After all, it's a great old model. Let's hope it's here to stay.

REMEMBER

If you have or suspect medical problems, don't go on a diet without consulting with your doctor first.

The best way to lose weight is to eat less and exercise more. Do that gradually and in moderation; don't eat a lot less and don't exercise a lot more without allowing your body to adjust.

Avoid fad diets; some are dangerous or at best useless. They may work for a while but the weight returns.

When you eat less, don't unbalance your diet. The best way is to follow the NutriScore system and select the foods you like from each area to reach the levels specified for those trying to lose weight, not more and not less.

Exercise regularly and build more physical activity such as walking and cycling into your daily routine.

Remember that it took years to put on weight. Taking it off should be slow and gradual. Once you reach your goal, adjust your diet with NutriScore, keep exercising and stay active. Then, you won't put all that weight back on again!

Chapter 4

Calorie-Maker
Number One: Fats

To run efficiently, the human body requires a certain number of calories per day (depending on age, size and sex), 30 per cent coming from fat, 60 per cent from carbohydrate and 10 per cent from protein. Upset this balance and the works go out of kilter: what should be a Rolls Royce becomes a jerky jalopy, operating on too much oil, not enough gas, and no anti-freeze at all.

Only laboratory analysis of our foods can tell if they have exactly the right proportions of calories and fat. Such analyses have been done. Scientists have charted the various values of almost all our foods. All we need is their charts to consult, the ability to add, and the sense to call it quits when the number of calories and the balance of fats, proteins and carbohydrates is right for the day.

Everybody needs some fat. In fact, 30 per cent of our daily calories should come from fat. The body requires this supply for its constant manufacture of living cells; it needs fats combined with proteins to line the intestines, to sheath nerve cells, even to make brain tissue.

Pork crackling and cream puffs don't go directly to your hips. The body breaks down the fat we eat, most of which is composed of glycerol and fatty acids from fats or carbohydrates, except for three essential fatty acids which are linoleic, linolenic, and arachidonic acids. Of these three, linoleic is the most important because, in a crunch, the body will make the others. They have to be in our foods. They are found in corn oil, sunflower seed, safflower, soybean and cottonseed oil. Our need for these fatty acids is small, which is why we seldom suffer any deficiency. Breast-fed babies are fortunate, since breast milk contains these three essential fatty acids. A baby on a formula lacking these essential fatty acids might experience the appearance of an exematous rash all over the body.

Fats are stored by the body in order to have a ready source of energy. They are held in the adipose tissue, which lies under the skin at various points, particularly around the abdomen. Adipose tissue cells have the remarkable ability of expanding to four or five times their normal size to accommodate more and more fat. When emptied they collapse somewhat but they never go away completely.

On some people fat seems here to stay, despite a conscientious diet and sufficient exercise. It could well be due to a large number of fat cells, which even when half filled remain sizable. So with the extra pounds gone, the cells remain, taking up space and, what's worse, lying in wait to trap any extra fat produced in the future. It hardly seems fair, but cells developed as early as our first year can plague us all our lives, as many erstwhile bouncing babies could testify, enroute to their diet workshops.

We know a family with two daughters who were brought up and fed alike, except during the crucial first year. The older girl was born in Northern Ireland, where plumpness was often equated with good health. Mother couldn't help comparing her slender child with the round, robust-looking babies at the infant clinic, and although the pediatrician said, "Not to worry," she started pushing cereals and rosehip syrup. At six months she was rewarded with compliments about the "beautiful big baby," but at twelve months, when they were back in Canada, comments like, "Look at little chubby-cheeks!" didn't sound quite so complimentary. She tried to limit her daughter's caloric intake from then on, but while the girl never became out-and-out fat, she stayed "chubby." Eventually, teenage vanity made the girl reduce, but it took real effort. Now, she's resigned to dieting for the rest of her life, because the least indulgence starts those fat cells puffing up again. Meanwhile, her younger sister who was not overfed in her first year of life has stayed slimmer. Even the occasional fling does not affect her figure and she will never be heavy enough to wear her sister's cast-off clothes.

The lowdown on the big three: cholesterol, saturates and polyunsaturates are the words most frequently heard these days in connection with fats and oils.

Cholesterol is one to get straight first. Cholesterol is a fat manufactured by our bodies. (There is also cholesterol in animal foods, because animals, like us, make their own.) Normally, cholesterol floats in the bloodstream, but when we manufacture too much it begins to collect in globs along the walls of our arteries, at times blocking the circulation, which results in a stroke or a heart attack. It is a wise preventive measure to limit the amount of cholesterol our body produces. Since the body uses the fatty acids with high hydrogen content (saturates) to make cholesterol, we can limit its production by avoiding this type of fat and eating more fats with low hydrogen content (polyunsaturates).

All fats, solid or liquid, are composed of glycerol and fatty acid molecules; the hydrogen's function is to fill in, or *saturate*, the gaps in the fatty acid molecules. Some molecules contain much more hydrogen than others. The effect of hydrogen is to turn the fat into a solid. We call these hydrogen-filled, solid fats *saturated fats*. Any solid fat, like butter, margarine, lard, or meat fat is saturated.

The unsaturated fats have fatty acid molecules with many gaps that have not been filled with hydrogen. These unfilled or *polyunsaturated fats* are equally simple to recognize because they come in the form of oils: corn oil, soybean oil, peanut oil, sunflower seed oil, safflower seed oil, and cottonseed oil. (Coconut and palm oils are a misnomer. They are saturated enough to be fats.)

Polyunsaturated fats are like a nutritional Drano. That's a bit extreme, but even supposing your arteries are somewhat gummed up at present, remember that the body is in a constant state of renovation. If you start using oil in place of butter or margarine, when the time comes to replace those cholesterol deposits, supplies will be unusually low. Better still, of course, is to prevent any buildup in the first place. The technique is to cut down on saturated fats. Stick to polyunsaturates; they won't stick to you.

Butter vs "the other spread." Butter is a saturated fat. For a while we were urged to give it up completely in favor of margarine, but recent research suggests butter may be the lesser of two evils.

Margarine has two things wrong with it. The first is that it is saturated fat. In order to solidify the oil to make margarine, manufacturers must set up specific conditions of temperature and pressure, employ a catalyst, and finally bubble into the prepared oil... hydrogen. Presto! Polyunsaturated oil becomes saturated margarine. It is true that the hydrogenation process stops much earlier with soft margarine, leaving it less saturated than butter or regular margarine, but the second objection to margarine applies to the soft variety as well as to the hard. Researchers now suspect that an undesirable chemical change occurs during margarine processing.

Trans-form fatty acids may develop as margarine is being made. The normal shape of a fatty acid molecule is one that is folded upon itself. That is the cis-form. The abnormal trans-form is a molecule that is stretched out. Scientists have long suspected that the stretched transform fatty acid molecule carries more cholesterol into the bloodstream and experiments at the University of Illinois appear to confirm this.

Dr. Fred A. Kummerow and his colleagues fed saturated fats like beef tallow and butter to certain baby pigs, polyunsaturated corn oil to others, and polyunsaturated margarine with 50 per cent trans-form fatty acids to a final group. The pigs receiving the trans-fatty acids developed the highest bloodfat levels and the highest blood-cholesterol levels, had the highest cholesterol deposits in their aortas, and showed more atherotic lesions in their aortas than did the other pigs.

If this is any indication of what humans can expect from margarine, maybe we'd better limit our use of it until all the facts are in. The only problem is, what to use for spreading and greasing and baking? Here's our solution.

May we present . . . a simple recipe.

BLENDED BUTTER

Makes ¾ pound (340 g)

Ingredients

2 tablespoons (25 mL) powdered skim milk

⅔ cup (150 mL) safflower oil (if unavailable, use sunflower, corn or soybean)

¼ pound (125 mL) butter at room temperature

Method

Using a blender or food processor is simpler than preparing the butter by hand. We have friends, however, who would rather spend the few minutes beating the mixture by hand than wash up after using the electric machines. It doesn't really matter. Whichever way you choose, the preparation is simple.

Combine milk powder and oil and allow them to sit together for 15 minutes or until the powder has softened. Add the butter and whip until thoroughly combined. Pour into a crock or other container and refrigerate.

Blended butter, for spreading, should be removed from the refrigerator just before use, as it softens rapidly at room temperature. The texture does not affect the taste, however. One of our testers whose finicky children always detected (and spurned) margarine was afraid that blended butter sandwiches might taste oily after a morning in a school locker. To her surprise the children didn't distinguish them from sandwiches made with pure butter. When she confessed to them what it was, they were so intrigued with the formula that they blended the next batch themselves.

To fancy up the spread a bit for use on French bread or fish or vegetables, try minced chives, parsley, lemon juice—you name it. Blended butter is soft enough that it's the work of a moment to stir in any flavor you like.

For baking, blended butter creams beautifully and can be substituted exactly for butter or margarine in cookies, cakes, coffee cakes, and quick breads. If your recipe calls for butter or margarine, replace the fat with an equal amount of blended butter and feel virtuous, but don't eat too much.

For frying and sautéing clarified blended butter has fewer ingredients still. Omit the milk powder. It adds to the spread's solidity, but since the butter is to be melted in any case, and is clarified beforehand, there is no milky residue.

Here is the recipe for making clarified blended butter.
Heat ¼ pound (125 mL) of butter until it liquifies. The milky residue will sink to the bottom and the clear, yellow liquid can be poured off to be later mixed with oil.
Remove from heat.
Add ¾ cup (175 mL) of safflower oil to the butter and beat well with a fork. Pour into a container and refrigerate.

The secret of any easy conversion to blended butter is to keep up your supplies. Buy ½ pound (225 g) of butter and use half for the spread and half for clarified blended butter. When they are half gone make up the next batch. Pretty soon it's automatic, like always keeping ahead with the frozen orange juice or the ice-cube tray.

The P/S ratio is the gauge we used to determine when we had developed a sufficiently healthful spread. P/S ratio means the amount of polyunsaturated fat (P) in comparison with the amount of saturated fat (S). To achieve a good P/S ratio a food must contain as much or slightly more polyunsaturates than saturates. We found that the highest practicable ratio for a fatty spread was around 1/1. Go much lower and there is too much saturated fat, but go much higher and it is oily and doesn't spread well. Butter, for example, has a P/S ratio of less than 0.1/1 which is far too low, but it does spread well. Safflower oil, has the excellent P/S ratio of approximately 7/1 but is awfully sloppy. Blended butter combines the two for a healthful ratio of about 1/1.

You may have wondered why we offer a choice of oils. Safflower oil has the best P/S ratio but is also the most expensive and hardest to find. Here is a chart showing the P/S ratios of the various oils and other fats on our shelves, so you can decide for yourself which best suits your purposes.

Watch out for palm oil and coconut oil. Their P/S ratio is terrible. The trouble is you probably eat them without knowing it, especially coconut oil, which is widely used in processed food.

Coconut oil is cheap. It doesn't feel greasy in snack foods like potato chips and cheesies. It browns to a very pleasing color, too, and is often

Comparison of Nutritional Quality of
Vegetable Oils in Relation to Their
P/S Ratio

Oil	P/S Ratio
Safflower oil	7/1
Sunflower oil	4/1
Corn oil	3/1
Soybean oil	3/1
Cottonseed oil	2/1
Peanut oil	1/1

sprayed on commercially baked cookies to make them appealingly golden. Finally, it doesn't go rancid when the food is dehydrated. This is why coconut oil is used in formulating cake and cookie mixes, synthetic coffee whiteners, whipped toppings, instant breakfasts, milkshake mixes, crackers, and ice cream coatings. We have no way of knowing whether these products actually contain coconut oil, because all the manufacturer is required to put on the label is "vegetable oil." The place you won't find coconut oil for certain is in cooking or salad oils. They are liquid at room temperature, and coconut oil is a "brittle" oil, which means it hardens at room temperature.

You will find coconut oil at the cosmetic counter, in face creams and shampoos, but as long as you keep them on the surface they'll do no harm.

Dare I eat a sterol or a phospholipid? Food contains other fatty substances, such as sterols and phospholipids, and since both of these are mentioned frequently in nutrition discussions, we'd better explain them here.

Cholesterol is a sterol found in certain animal foods like eggs, liver, kidney, and shellfish. These foods also contain such excellent nutrients as protein, vitamins A and B, and iron. The question arises whether we should sacrifice their nutritional value in order to avoid their cholesterol.

We think the answer is no. Used in moderation foods such as eggs and liver have many benefits and will not affect the blood level of cholesterol seriously, which is what counts. The trick is to give your body only as much cholesterol as it can handle effectively.

How do you tell on a day-to-day basis when you've reached the exact level of cholesterol the body can handle without increasing the amount

Cholesterol Content of Foods

Food	Size of Serving		Cholesterol (mg)
Beef, cooked	3 oz.	(85 g)	80
Butter	½ cup	(125 mL)	280
Butter	1 tbsp.	(15 mL)	30
Butter	1 pat	(5 mL)	10
Cheese, Cheddar	1 oz.	(30 g)	30
Cheese, cottage	½ cup	(125 mL)	20
Cheese, cream	1 oz.	(30 mL)	30
Cheese, spread	1 oz.	(30 mL)	30
Chicken, cooked (flesh only)	3 oz.	(85 g)	70
Crab, in shell (meat only)	3 oz.	(85 g)	100
Egg, whole	1	(50 g)	270
Fish, steak, cooked	3 oz.	(85 g)	60
Fish, fillet, cooked	3 oz.	(85 g)	60
Heart, cooked	3 oz.	(85 g)	170
Ice cream	1 cup	(250 mL)	60
Kidney	3 pieces	(55 g)	420
Lamb, cooked	3 oz.	(85 g)	80
Lard	1 cup	(250 mL)	500
Lard	1 tbsp.	(15 mL)	30
Liver, cooked	2 oz.	(55 g)	200
Lobster, meat only	3 oz.	(85 g)	220
Margarine, all veg.	½ cup	(125 mL)	0
Milk, fluid, whole	1 cup	(250 mL)	30
Milk, fluid, skim	1 cup	(250 mL)	0
Oysters, raw (meat only)	1 cup	(250 mL)	480
Pork, cooked	3 oz.	(85 g)	80
Shrimp, in shell, (flesh only)	1 cup	(250 mL)	180
Sweetbreads	3½ oz.	(100 g)	250
Veal, cooked	3 oz.	(85 g)	100

in the blood? On the basis of scientific findings we can offer you a rule of thumb. If you keep your fat intake down and have as little of it as possible in saturated form, you can afford to eat about 350 mg of cholesterol per day or 2500 mg per week. Considering that an egg contains 270 mg of cholesterol and that there are only 200 mg in a two-ounce serving of liver, you can see that it is not necessary to deprive yourself of these very nourishing foods. Three eggs and a serving of

liver each week will have only 1000 mg, leaving you with 1500 mg of cholesterol to go. At present the average cholesterol intake in North America is between 600 and 800 mg per day or about 5000 mg per week, which is about twice what it should be. The following table gives the cholesterol content of some common and healthful foods. Choose your favorite 350 mg, limit your fats, and enjoy yourself.

Lecithin is a phospholipid found mainly in eggs and in seeds such as soybean. It is an emulsifying agent that prevents oil and water from separating and is used for this purpose in many processed foods. It does nobody any harm. On the other hand, it performs no magic, either. Lecithin does *not* dissolve cholesterol deposits in the blood stream, as some health food proponents claim. All the lecithin we can use is manufactured in our own bodies. When an outside supply arrives in the form of food or pills, the body breaks it down and either burns it for energy or excretes it in the urine. So don't waste hard-earned money on lecithin capsules; put it instead into safflower oil that *will* help lower your cholesterol.

Keep your balance: a maximum of 30 per cent of your daily calories should come from fat. We've said it before and we'll say it again.

What foods have the most fat? If 30 per cent of your calories are budgeted for fat, you'll want to spend that 30 per cent wisely. On page 48 is a chart that lists foods in terms of the proportion of calories coming from fat.

If you eat foods around the 30 per cent mark you are right on. If you choose foods too far above that mark, make sure that some are also below so that it will even out. For example, peanut butter is 76 per cent fat calories while bread is 11 per cent fat calories. When you combine them in a peanut butter sandwich, you have a reasonable level of 44 per cent fat calories. Don't forget amounts make a difference, too. Peanut butter spreads thickly or thinly. There are also instances where you are better off substituting one food for another. Drink whole milk at 50 per cent fat calories. Or, better yet, drop it and pick skim milk at 0 per cent. As you plan a meal or a snack, at home or in a restaurant, think about the chart. It can help you avoid overdrawing the fat account.

Don't give up anything, just cut down. If most of your favorite foods showed up on the chart as being over 50 per cent fat, clearly you'll have to take some action to preserve your health. But don't swear off bologna forever, because it won't work. If you love a food and have been accustomed to it since childhood, sudden deprivation is too hard—you'll probably wind up having a bologna binge. Recognize instead that it has a lot of fat, and then tell yourself you can have a

Percentage of Calories from Fat in Foods

Over 50%

Cream cheese
Weiners
Peanuts and peanut butter
Pork lunch meats
Most cheese and cheese spreads
Tongue
Eggs
Ground beef—regular
Salmon, tuna (canned in oil)
Pork—loin and butt
Granola

50%

Chicken—roasted, flesh and skin
Beef—porterhouse, T-bone, round
    rump, lean ground, kidney
Pork—fresh and cured ham and
    shoulder
Lamb—shoulder, rib
Salmon—red sockeye, canned

Whole milk
Ice cream
Cream cheese
    sandwich
Peanut butter
    sandwich

30%

Beef—sirloin, arm, flank, heart
Turkey—flesh and skin, dark meat
Lamb—leg, loin
Pork—heart, kidney
Chicken—dark meat, roasted flesh

Creamed cottage
    cheese
Lunch meat or
Cheese spread
    sandwich

40%

Beef—heel of round, pot roast
Liver—pork, chicken, lamb, beef
Fish—bass, ciscoe, oysters, salmon (pink)
Chicken—roasted, light meat broilers—no skin

20%

Under 20%

Fish—haddock, cod, tuna, (water pack) ocean perch, halibut,
    smelt, sole
Shellfish—most
Porridge
Bread
Most peas, beans, and lentils
Skin milk cheese
Uncreamed cottage cheese
Skim milk
Most breakfast cereals (other than granola type)

bologna sandwich on fish days but not on steak days. Eat a little less this week and next week a little less and after that a little less. . . .

Some foods are fat but good for you. Take canned salmon—it's in the 60 or 70 per cent fat range, but it also contains protein, vitamins, minerals, and a calcium bonus (or it should be bone-us, since processing transfers calcium from the bones to the meat and juice of the salmon). Make a salmon casserole from a can of salmon, incorporating its juice in the sauce, and you'll have bought a lot of good nutrition with your fat calories, and a good, fairly cheap meal.

Or take peanut butter. Either you love it or you hate it, but acknowledge its value as a protein source. One tablespoonful (15 mL) makes a nourishing, not too fat or fattening sandwich.

For another high fat food with enough nourishment to make it worth a chunk of your 30 per cent fat calories, eat an egg . . . but not too often. Each egg is 60 to 70 per cent fat calories, so it should be eaten in moderation for the high-quality protein, iron, vitamins and minerals it contains, say three or four a week.

You can figure out for yourself from the fat-content chart plus information elsewhere in the book whether a high fat food has enough other things going for it to deserve a place in your menu. Just one hint: When you're choosing meat remember the fat-content chart, and when you do, remember that as far as cutting down fat content goes, the food at the bottom is tops.

To cook lean, learn our seven steps to fearless frying: cook in advance. Let the fat congeal on top and then throw it out. This doesn't apply when you have an oven roast of beef, pork, or lamb, but it does when you're making stew, or pot roast, or braised shoulder, or any meat dish to which you add liquid. Cook slowly, refrigerate when cool, and that night or the next day—or even a couple of days later—lift off the hardened fat. If you've never tried day-after stew you're in for a nice surprise. It tastes richer than fresh-off-the-stove stew, and you'll be amazed at the amount of fat congealed on top. That should go into the garbage and not into you. The same trick works for spaghetti or barbecue sauces. Make them on the weekend and you'll be set come woeful Wednesday.

Make greaseless gravy. Drain the roast and pop the pan juices into the freezer. Remove the solidified fat and reheat the juices as is or blend them with two tablespoons (25 mL) of flour per cup (250 mL) of meat juice, and heat, stirring until the gravy is creamy smooth.

Don't be a browner. We've found that casseroles of chicken, turkey, meat, or whatever are flavorful without browning the meat beforehand. So don't brown; just mix the meat, vegetables and other ingredients and head for the stove. It's a two for one bargain; you save on fat calories and avoid dirty pans at the same time.

If you ever brown foods, use butter or animal shortening, so that the fat will congeal when the dish is chilled. Oil won't congeal and therefore can't be chucked in the garbage. The time to use oil for browning is if you are making something like onion soup to be used right after cooking. Since you must brown the onions and eat the fat, use a polyunsaturated fat such as corn oil.

Frying fat-free. It is fool-proof. With the new non-stick pans, such as T-Fal and SilverStone to name names, you can sauté onions, brown pancakes and scramble eggs without a soupçon of fat. Perfectionist chefs moan over the absence of the particles left on the pan necessary for the "de-glaze"; others rave about the health possibilities of fat-free cookery. Master chef Pierre Franey, now staff writer for the New York Times, wrote "they are of unquestioned value for those on special diets. An important contemporary use for these surfaces is in the preparation of some *nouvelle cuisine* dishes ... which are notable for using as little oil or butter as possible." He recommends, as we do, that you spend a little more to purchase a heavy aluminum pan coated with the newer materials and experiment with them for recipes that call for sautéing or pan frying. Here's a recipe for a low-calorie no-fat soup.

DIETER'S RATATOUILLE SOUP

Ratatouille is a traditional summer salad or vegetable dish made with eggplant, zucchini, tomatoes, and olive oil. This soup has the extravagant summer flavor and satisfying taste of ratatouille without the oil. 42 calories in all!

1 Serving
Ingredients
Fat-free prepared pan (trade names are Teflon, T-Fal, etc.)
2 tablespoons (25 mL) medium chopped onion
3 tablespoons (50 mL) cubed green or red pepper
½ cup (125 mL) or more cubed zucchini
½ cup (125 mL) or more cubed eggplant
¼ teaspoon (1 mL) minced hot pepper or pinch dried hot peppers
1 tablespoon (15 mL) minced parsley
¼ teaspoon (1 mL) garlic salt
pinch dried oregano
pinch freshly ground pepper
6 ounce (177 mL) can or ¾ cup (175 mL) vegetable juice

Method
This cold soup tastes best if the flavors are allowed to blend for a day or two.
Heat the pan and add the onion, stirring to soften for about 1-2 minutes. Add pepper and stir. Add zucchini, hot pepper, and eggplant, cover and simmer over low heat for 4-5 minutes. Add parsley and seasonings, stir to blend. Add vegetable juice. Pour into a container and cover. Store in the refrigerator. When ready to serve, either as a lunch or a cold soup for a meal starter, garnish with a dollop of yogurt or a lemon slice.

For a low calorie meal:	Ratatouille soup	42 calories
	Rye crackers, 4	46 calories
	Yogurt, 6 oz. (175 mL)	112 calories
	With sliced fruit	
	(e.g., 1 medium peach)	35 calories
		235 calories

Give 'em the bird. Fowl is a terrific several-times-a-week food, because it's flavorful and versatile and down at the lean end of the list, particularly if you skin it. Look at the comparison:

Fowl	*% fat calories with skin*	*% fat calories without skin*
Roast chicken	53	31
Roast turkey	39	29
Roast goose	78	38

Remove the skin from roast fowl after cooking, but try skinning smaller pieces before you cook them. If you're using a sauce you can extract further fat by cooking as usual, refrigerating, removing the congealed fat and reheating.

Spring or young chickens and turkeys are the leanest.

Type	*Weight*	*% fat calories with skin*
Broilers or fryers	small (1½-2½ lbs. or about 1 kg)	37
Roasters	medium (2½-4½ lbs. or 1-2 kg)	63
Stewing hens	fat, mature (2-5½ lbs. or 1-2.5 kg)	78

As you can see from the chart, by buying young fowl and/or skinning and skimming it you can easily serve low-fat chicken and turkey dinners. You can also fatten it up by greasing the skin with butter and serving the chicken with skin, dressing, and gravy but believe us, it isn't necessary. Part of the pleasure of fowl lies in the delicate taste; don't mask it!

Cure your fatty frypan—Sauté onions without fat, you hear? Impossible, you say. Aha, it isn't so. Instead of fat, try 1 or 2 tablespoons (15 to 25 mL) of chicken stock to sauté those onions and peppers. Granted, the stock doesn't lift and hold the flavor as well as fat, but it is quite passable—and in terms of health, exceptional. Here's a recipe to try . . . and by the way, there's a saving of 70 to 100 calories using our "cure" and few would notice the difference.

CHICKEN LIVERS WITH VEGETABLES

Serve it with a side salad of lettuce, dressed with lemon or tomato yogurt dressing.

1 Serving
The pieces of liver and pieces of vegetable should be cut the same size and shape.

Ingredients
1 tablespoon (15 mL) chicken broth
½ medium onion, cut in quarters
½ green pepper, cut in eighths
¼ pound (115 g) chicken livers, cleaned and halved
2 teaspoons (10 mL) Worcestershire sauce
½ tomato, seeded and cut in quarters

Method
Heat a small sauté or fry pan, large enough to hold the vegetables and livers. Add broth. Add onion and cook lightly until soft—about 3-4 minutes. Add pepper, livers and sauce and sauté lightly, turning them until the livers have turned brown. Cover and cook on simmer heat for 3-4 minutes. Add tomatoes and heat for about 2 minutes. Remove the livers and vegetables to a plate to keep warm and boil the gravy to reduce it until there are 2 tablespoons (25 mL) left. Pour over dish and serve.

Calories: 70 calories in each serving (% calories from fat = 0) For a low calorie meal: *Calories*

	Calories
Lettuce salad	10
Dressing of chopped tomato and yogurt	20
Chicken livers with vegetables	70
Sliced pineapple, fresh or packed in its own juice ½ cup (125 mL)	40
Total Calories =	140

Check the oil. Oil is fat, and adds to the day's fat calories. Oils have the desirable quality of having a good P/S ratio. (Remember, the more polyunsaturates the better.) So, as much as possible make your fat the right kind of oil. Safflower oil is best, but when you can't find it or afford it, corn, sunflower, soybean, and cottonseed oils are good for salads. The blended butter on page 43 is best for spreading, cooking and baking.

What fat to use when? The rule is oil (polyunsaturated, of course) whenever you can. However, here's a chart to help in deciding what to use:

Spreading	Baking	Pan Frying
Blended butter	Blended butter for cookies or butter cakes.	Oil for a dish not cooked in sauce to be eaten immediately
	(You can make blended lard as you make blended butter only substitute lard for butter to lower cost.)	Butter or lard if you have to brown before cooking. Remove fat after chilling.
	Oil for muffins, loaves and pastry (for pastry recipes— see Chapter 16)	

REMEMBER

To live off the fat of the land means to have the best of everything, and what's wrong with that? The best fat should come from the bottom of the fat-content chart more often than from the top and should add up to 30 per cent of your daily calories. If you follow these guidelines, you will look and feel as if you have lived *off* the fat, not just stored it.

How can you tell if a food has too much fat? Easily. If you can see fat or feel its richness in your mouth, the food has too much fat.

You should favor the polyunsaturated (the fluid ones like vegetable oils) over the saturated fats (the solid ones like animal fat) to cut down your cholesterol. But, don't be fooled by coconut and palm oils—they are saturated enough to be solid fats.

You can now solve the age-old "butter or margarine" controversy. Try the blended butter recipe. It is easy to make and gives you less saturates and more polyunsaturates than butter alone would.

Foods that are high in cholesterol also tend to be rich in vitamins, minerals, and protein. Rather than cut them out, cut them down. Be satisfied with three or four eggs and a serving of liver every week. That much you will need.

There are many ways to cut down on fat in your food. Choose skim milk and skim-milk cheese instead of whole milk and cream cheese.

Follow our seven steps: Cook ahead; Make greaseless gravy; Skim your stews; Skin your fowl; Fry fat-free; Simmer your sautés; and check your oil—make sure it is polyunsaturated.

Chapter 5

Calorie-Maker
Number Two: Carbohydrates

Carbohydrates have an undeservedly bad reputation. Think about it. Which two foods do people most commonly give up when the pounds accumulate? Do we hear bread and potatoes? The teenager lunching on ham between slices of cheese, the business man doubling his portion of steak in order to forgo baked potato, and the housewife serving strange unappetizing protein combinations are all trying to avoid carbohydrates—for no good reason, and sometimes with unfortunate results. The ridiculous, uncritical publicity given to the recent plague of low-carbohydrate, high-fat diets implies we can drastically reduce our carbohydrate intake without consequences. Nonsense. Dangerous nonsense. For proper nutrition you should aim at getting 60 per cent of your daily calories in the form of carbohydrates.

The balance of nutrients that you achieve by rating at the desirable levels in all areas in NutriScore gives you the carbohydrates you need. They are mainly in foods listed in areas C, D, F, and G. Of course, some are in foods in area H, and these we like to discourage because these foods are so refined that the carbohydrates are mainly in the form of sugar and contain few to no vitamins, minerals, or proteins.

There is an appalling amount of misinformation concerning carbohydrates: from the rumor that they are unnecessary to the myth that sugar gives instant energy. Here are some solid facts.

What are carbohydrates? Carbohydrates are starches and sugars. They are found in such foods as bread, cereals, potatoes, pastas, rice, fruits, vegetables, milk, ice cream and yogurt. Not only do these carbohydrates combine with other nutrients that are essential to our health but they are themselves essential in providing energy to the body and in particular to the muscles and the brain.

The body digests carbohydrates first. When we eat a meal the last thing to be digested are fats, the second last are proteins and the first to be digested are the carbohydrates. Carbohydrates are easily broken down into simple sugars that are turned into the blood sugar, glucose.

Glucose is carried by the bloodstream to provide energy for all parts of the body. In hospital, when a patient cannot utilize any other form of nourishment, his energy is preserved and his system is kept functioning by means of a glucose solution. Glucose maintains the premature baby until it is strong enough to drink and it gives the person undergoing an operation sustenance until it is safe for him to take normal meals. At that stage the post-operative invalid will be offered a high-carbohydrate diet because it is simplest and quickest for his body to use and will help him build up the energy to absorb proteins and fats later on. Far from being unnecessary, carbohydrates are essential.

We can only store a small amount of carbohydrates. If the blood receives more glucose than it and the rest of the body require at that time, a small amount of the excess is turned into a starch called glycogen and stored in the liver and muscles. The maximum glycogen storage is equivalent to about 600 calories.

Carbohydrates make us fat only when we eat more than we need. When we eat more carbohydrates than the blood and body require in the form of glucose and more than can be stored in the form of glycogen, then the excess is converted to fat and is stored in the fat cells of the adipose tissue. It is not carbohydrates but overeating that makes us fat.

Fats and proteins make us fat, too. If the body receives too much fat, it simply stores the extra. If the body gets more protein than it needs, it converts the protein first to carbohydrates, and subsequently to fat which it stores. Extra calories are extra calories and they make us fat, in whatever form.

If we are short of carbohydrates can our bodies burn fat and protein for energy? Yes, but to a limited extent. Fat can be used as a direct source of energy and protein can form glucose and glycogen, which provides energy for the brain and muscles.

Isn't this a good way to get rid of excess fat? No. Fat is not a favorite source of energy for our mental and physical powerhouses, the brain and muscles. They prefer blood sugar (glucose) as their source of energy and, lacking carbohydrates, the body has to provide it by breaking down some of its protein. It is certainly not desirable to destroy the protein the body needs for the proper functioning of such vital parts as the immune system, which protects us from disease and infection. You may wonder why you can't increase protein at the very moment of cutting down on carbohydrates, so that the protein can be utilized for glucose production directly. First, your timing would have to be pretty close to balance different rates of digestion. Also, it would be a dangerous way to treat the kidneys, because they would have to bear the unaccustomed burden of discharging the debris left from changing large amounts of protein into glucose. If you have ever tried a high-protein diet, you'll remember how much water you were urged to drink and how much time was spent flushing out your overworked kidneys.

No part of the body operates in a vacuum. Every function is dependent on, or contributes to, some other function. If you are fortunate enough to have a smoothly running system, it is foolhardy to short circuit any part of it. Better to short circuit your trips to the refrigerator, and keep your meals small and balanced.

Some people are diabetics; they can't handle carbohydrates. To find out if you are a diabetic or likely to become one, examine your family history. Diabetes is often inherited. Watch for certain symptoms. A diabetic initially notices that he is thirsty all the time and urinates frequently and eats a lot. As the disease develops the symptoms include blurred vision, skin irritation, muscle weakness, and coma. If there is a family history of diabetes or you have the initial symptoms, consult your physician and seek the help of a nutritionist through your doctor.

Diabetes results from a shortage of insulin, a hormone that we produce every time we eat carbohydrates. Insulin helps the tissues extract the sugar from the blood. In the absence of insulin, blood sugar stays in the blood and gets lost in the urine without the body using it. This has devastating effects.

If the condition is mild, the answer is to consume a small amount of carbohydrates, enough to match the body's capacity. If the condition is severe it will be necessary to take insulin injections. Your doctor and nutritionist will work it out for you.

But then, there are hypoglycemics. They have the opposite condition. Their bodies produce too much insulin. Their tissues just slurp sugar and the blood sugar level drops severely. In simple terms, hypoglycemia is a blood sugar deficiency.

Normally the body is equipped with a fine insulin control mechanism. The sugar we eat pours into the blood and the insulin tap is turned on, signalling the muscles and other tissue to use the blood sugar or store it as glycogen. When we eat starch, the blood isn't flooded with sugar, because it takes time to digest the starch, and the sugar from the starch is absorbed slowly. So, the insulin tap comes on gradually.

Possibly, the frequent eating of sugar, such as in candy, soft drinks, sweetened coffee or tea, puts a strain on the insulin tap. The controls, which should be finely regulated, can become sluggish. For some people the insulin comes on and doesn't shut off fast enough; the result is hypoglycemia.

The symptoms of hypoglycemia are easy to recognize. They are also easy to imagine. So, if you suspect the condition, go to your doctor and have a glucose tolerance test. Here is what you will notice if you are hypoglycemic: at first, there is a feeling of emptiness (not hunger), fatigue, irritability, and tightness in the chest with shallow breathing. This may be accompanied by dizziness and attacks of sweating with rapid and audible heart beats. In some people these symptoms are accompanied by headaches. The symptoms occur about three hours after a meal and are relieved by eating. The question is what to eat. If you take a sugar tablet (as some advocate), a candy, or a soft drink, you will raise the blood sugar level and relieve the symptoms temporarily. Eating sugar will also turn on the insulin tap in full. So, you may be better off eating starch as in bread, biscuits, muffins, or protein as in cheese, meat, beans, peanut butter, and eggs. The relief might be slower but another attack might be avoided. The most important thing to remember if you are hypoglycemic is *never to skip a meal*. You need all your meals and you need them moderate in size and evenly spaced. If you can cut down on the amount you eat at mealtime, you can plan a nutritious snack mid-morning, mid-afternoon, and midnight. Borrow a muffin from your breakfast, an apple or a slice of cheese from your lunch, and a glass of milk from your dinner. You should also watch for certain foods that are reputed to trigger a flow of insulin and precipitate an attack. Coffee and alcohol are known to do just that for some people. Try decaffeinated coffee or tea and certainly moderate or eliminate your liquor consumption. Whatever you do, never drink alcohol on an empty stomach; always have something to eat when you drink.

Hypoglycemia has been the platform for many health quacks. There is a proliferation of books, magazine articles, and TV and radio interviews warning us about our blood sugar. At the same time, the medical establishment dismisses the whole issue as one of little importance, repeating that there are very few cases of hypoglycemia. It could be that many hypoglycemics suffer in ignorance or treat themselves without medical help. If you suspect you are hypoglycemic, find out. Your doctor can examine you and diagnose your condition. If you are hypoglycemic, insist on a consultation with a nutritionist to get the do's and the don'ts straight.

What does alcohol do to you? It does a lot to you and for you. Alcohol is a simple chemical with a structure similar to that of sugar. It is not normally formed in the body. Being a small molecule, alcohol moves easily into the blood and changes the structure of the blood components. So the body has to burn it fast since it can't get rid of it in the urine. The only organ that can handle alcohol is the liver. If it becomes overloaded, alcohol concentration in the blood will rise and some of it will get into the brain (making you giddy) and into the lungs and your breath, a sure way to fail a breathalyzer test. In the liver, alcohol is burned and transformed into calories. From one ounce (30 mL) of alcohol you get around 150 calories (more than what you get from an ounce of carbohydrate or protein, but less than from an ounce of fat).

In order for the liver to burn alcohol, certain enzymes must work efficiently, which they can do only with the aid of protein and certain vitamins and minerals. This is why, if you are going to drink, you'll have to eat a balanced diet. The body has to be well nourished. But for heavy drinkers the paradox is that all too often they neglect to eat properly. Some may eat a lot, but not a nutritionally balanced diet.

Excessive drinking beyond the ability of the liver to burn alcohol leads to a pathological condition called cirrhosis of the liver, which can be fatal.

One never starts out as a heavy drinker. Social drinkers can drift into alcoholism without realizing it. It creeps up on many of us. So, it is important to be on guard not to become dependent on drinking alcohol.

Alcoholism is a state of addictive need to consume large amounts of alcohol regularly. "Large" could be defined as six or more 1¼ oz. (35 mL) shots of liquor, or 5 oz. (150 mL) glasses of wine, or 12 oz. bottles of beer (341 mL) per day, although it must be pointed out that for persons whose liver cannot handle much alcohol the effects of alcohol are achieved with smaller quantities.

If you are a habitual drinker, regardless of how few drinks you take per day, you should test your ability to abstain for two or more consecutive days without suffering any irritability or other withrawal symptoms.

Excessive drinking can ruin your health. In the first place, alcohol is nothing but empty calories and it all too often replaces food containing the protein, vitamins, and minerals that we need to function properly. The food calories it spares could lead to obesity and coronary heart disease. What's more, alcohol interferes with the absorption of several B vitamins and deprives the body of these vitamins even when they are in the diet.

Alcohol disrupts normal sleep and exercise patterns. It slowly interferes with the normal function of the brain, and could lead to fatal liver disease.

It takes time for the body to convert sugar into energy. There goes the old idea of sugar as an instant energy food. The swimmer downing a dixie cup of corn syrup while she floats won't reap the benefit at the next wave. On the other side of the lake, yes, but the energy she's using now comes from food she ate earlier. It takes time for the sugar to be absorbed and to be picked up by the muscle and burned for energy.

An athlete needs all kinds of food, such as whole grains, fresh fruits, vegetables, and milk, to provide not only carbohydrates, but also many of the other nutrients needed to build a strong body. It is true, however, that an athlete's meal immediately before an athletic event should be readily digestible, and this means avoiding high-fat foods.

We don't need sugar if we have starch. It is true that we can do without sugar except for taste. We are all so accustomed to the taste of sugar that it is unrealistic to expect anyone not suffering from sugar-related medical problems such as diabetes to give it up entirely. In fact, it is practically impossible to give up because sugar forms a part of many everyday products—soups, condiments, and cereals. You probably eat more than you think you do; it is estimated that each of us consumes more than 100 pounds (45.36 kg) of sugar a year in prepared foods, in pies, cookies, cakes and beverages.

As for nutrition, sugar (be it raw or refined, in honey, or in syrup, or any of the sweeteners) has nothing to offer but carbohydrate calories. Medical evidence points to sugar as a prominent cause of dental caries and for some people it is a factor in heart disease as well. Sweeteners certainly contribute to obesity, since only one spoonful of sugar contains 25 calories, and they indirectly contribute to malnutrition by replacing more healthful foods. If apples and chocolate cake are available for dessert the cake-eaters don't usually have room for a nourishing apple as well. And how many times have you heard, "I'll have to skip breakfast to make up for all these brownies, but it's worth it"?

"Reducing Sugar." For both weight control and general health we should all cut back on the amount of sugar in our daily menu. Doing without is of course the best method, but even if you have a sweet tooth there are ways to eliminate sweets and never miss them.

Don't worry about the sugar you can't avoid. If you're hooked on ketchup, canned soup, pork and beans, barbecue sauce, and other items listing sugar on the label, recognize that they contain sugar and try to eat them in smaller amounts accompanied with unsweetened nourishing foods; but don't make yourself miserable, as long as these processed foods constitute only a small part of your diet.

Reduce the amount of sugar you add. You have the upper hand at the sugar canister. Make it a light hand for a lighter you. Here are some tricks we use to reduce sugar.

Use jelly or pectin-added jam because they contain less sugar, and spread them thinly on your peanut butter sandwich.

Cut in half the amount of sugar you add to beverages. If you take two teaspoons of sugar in coffee and average daily two cups at breakfast, one at coffee break, lunch, four o'clock and dinner time, plus one more spoonful on cereal or fruit or what have you, your sugar intake for the day will be 3½ ounces (100 grams). That's not counting the sugar used in cooking, either. So, if you cut out 3½ ounces (100 grams) of sugar per day you will eat 80 pounds (36.4 kg) less sugar a year. *After you've cut your sugar to half, try cutting it out entirely.*

And don't fall victim to the fructose fad. Fructose fanciers claim that it is the "no-sugar" sugar, or "low calorie" sugar or "good-for-diabetics" sugar, whereas it is really the other half of table sugar (glucose is the first half). It is found naturally in fruits and honey and is to be treated by diabetics in the same way as all sugars to be avoided.

Some researchers have found it to be slightly less likely to contribute to cavities than ordinary sugar; but others have found it to be the form of sugar most likely to change to cholesterol in the body. It is sweeter than either sucrose or glucose. If you have a sweet tooth, fructose is not the answer. Its sudden fame probably relates more to the fact that industry has now found a way to produce it more economically and in quantity than anything else.

Use sugar substitutes, such as saccharin, in moderation. There is a lot of talk at the present time concerning the use of sugar substitutes. We believe that in small amounts they are safe and helpful to the person who is accustomed to a sweet taste. But use them to help cut down on sweets, not to replace sweets. Don't teach your palate to demand large amounts of sweetness, non-caloric or otherwise.

Cut down on table sugar. Use the syrup from canned fruit for gelatin desserts. Some canned fruit is packed in syrup as rich as 45 per cent sugar. Serve the fruit drained and perhaps combined with yogurt and raisins as one dessert and make another with the syrup and softened dissolved plain gelatin. Follow the instructions on your gelatin package, using the fruit syrup as liquid. When it is partially set you could add sliced fresh fruit for extra nourishment. This way you get two desserts for the cost of one can of fruit and an inexpensive envelope of gelatin, and you use up the banana that was getting too ripe or the last of the berries.

Add raisins or other dried fruit to the water for hot cereal. They will plump up as the water boils and sweeten the cereal so that sugar is unnecessary. On a cold morning your family will consider it a treat.

Top unsugared whole-grain cold cereals with milk and a tablespoon (15 mL) of a sugared whole-grain cereal like Alpen or Shreddies. Mixing a slightly pre-sweetened cereal with one not sweetened at all could be the answer for many sweet-tooth families.

Stop sighing—say no. Too many times we get sweet-talked into doing what we don't want to do. They say the best defense is a good offense. So, in order to protect yourself and your family from poor health habits you may have to go on the attack. Learn to say: "No, I certainly won't buy that junk"; "No, Mother, I don't want the children to have candy every time you visit"; "No, dear, I want a walk, not a liqueur." Does it sound awful? Would you rather say, "Too bad, honey, but the dentist can't help hurting" or "How are we ever going to get twenty pounds off you?"

We don't mean you should be rigid. Of course, you'll still buy cookies from the family Brownie. Serve them for dessert that very day and pop the rest in the freezer until mid-summer when they'll be a special treat for visitors whose own cookies were eaten long ago. Let Grandma be the Easter bunny and maybe she'll bring comic books on ordinary Sundays. It's not the special occasions that count, it's the day-to-day intake of sweets that you want to regulate. To people who normally don't eat candy, one chocolate is enough.

We could live all our lives without sweetened baked goods, but on occasions like birthdays and for active growing children with "hollow legs" baking cakes and cookies may be unavoidable. The aim is to make them as low in sugar and as high in other nutrients as possible.

The less refined the food is the better. Instead of butter-frosted white cake, make a date and nut loaf. Instead of shortbread, make raisin squares and molasses oatmeal cookies.

Reduce the sugar in coffee cakes and cookies. If the recipe calls for one cup (250 mL) of sugar, use two-thirds of a cup (150 mL). If you find the texture, taste, and appearance just as good as before (and they probably will be), next time reduce the sugar a little further, maybe even to half. We have tried this reduction system in our test kitchen with the following typical results.

Butter cakes, sponge cakes, all types of sweet breads, muffins, and cookies were slightly lighter in color but just as tasty with two-thirds the sugar called for in the recipe. Even custards and puddings were as delicious as ever with less sugar. In some cases, the flavor was improved. Gingerbread and lemon sauce was more gingery and tart,— delicious. A standard butter cake was more delicate. Date squares and muffins had a lovely flavor that had been hidden before.

If you can't reduce the sugar, cut the trimmings. Angel food cake and meringue pie need the sugar to help hold the air and support them. They don't need chocolate sauce. A butter cake is rich enough without a creamy icing. Confectioners sugar sprinkled through a paper doily is an old-fashioned topping that gives an intricate lacy appearance. Children particularly like the design and find it quite sweet enough. For family eating stick to yeast fruit cakes, loaves, and breakfast breads and cookies.

Just passing through. There is a further reason why we should not eliminate carbohydrate foods from our diet. We need unrefined carbohydrate foods for their fiber. Fiber is what provides structure to a plant's leaves, stems, and fruits; it is to a plant what bones are to an animal. Fiber is made up of cellulose and other complex carbohydrates that are not broken down by our digestive enzymes. Thus, it remains a bulky material that helps mop out the debris remaining after digestion and absorption. It is fiber that adds volume and weight to fecal matter and facilitates its passage through the intestines.

Nutritionists have long advocated a certain amount of fiber in the diet. No available studies have determined what amount or type is necessary, but good digestion is associated with a diet containing large quantities of vegetables and fruits and unrefined cereals rather than large amounts of meat and refined cereals. Followers of high-protein, low-carbohydrate diets will tell you that infrequent bowel movements are one result of such diets.

Recent studies have suggested that fiber plays a role in the prevention of cancer of the colon and of heart disease. The interpretation of these studies is not clear-cut, because there are many variables besides diet which might account for differences. But it is clear that African populations consuming large quantities of fruits and vegetables and unrefined cereals do not suffer cancer of the colon as do Western populations consuming large quantities of meat and refined cereals. Also, populations on an unrefined diet, high in fiber, suffer fewer heart attacks than those on refined diets, low in fiber.

The stimulation of fecal movements in the absence of fiber is possible. Certain foods like prune juice have a laxative effect. Mineral oil is sometimes used to soften fecal matter and facilitate its movement. Whether these products aid in the prevention of disease is unknown. The repeated use of mineral oil, however, is undesirable because it causes massive excretion of the fat-soluble vitamins, such as A, D, E, and K.

Dietary Fiber Content of Foods

Food	Size of Serving		Fiber (g)
Fruit:			
Apples with skin	1	(150 g)	5
Apricots, stewed	4	(100 g)	9
Bananas	1	(175 g)	5
Figs, stewed	3	(100 g)	10
Oranges, peeled	1	(180 g)	4
Prunes, stewed	5	(100 g)	8
Raspberries	¾ cup	(175 mL)	7
Vegetables:			
Broccoli	½ cup	(125 mL)	1
Carrots, raw	1	(50 g)	1
Cauliflower	¾ cup	(175 mL)	3
Celery, raw	1	(40 g)	1
Corn, on the cob	1 ear	(140 g)	7
Leeks	4	(100 g)	3
Lentils, cooked	½ cup	(125 mL)	3
Lettuce	2 leaves	(50 g)	1
Peas, cooked	½ cup	(125 mL)	4
Spinach, boiled	½ cup	(125 mL)	6
Nuts:			
Almonds	¼ cup	(50 mL)	4
Peanuts	¼ cup	(50 mL)	4
Peanut butter	2 tbsp.	(25 mL)	2
Breads and Cereals:			
All Bran Cereal	½ cup	(125 mL)	7
Corn Flakes	1 cup	(250 mL)	2
Meusli	½ cup	(125 mL)	2
Puffed Wheat	1 cup	(250 mL)	2
Rice, boiled	½ cup	(125 mL)	2
Shredded Wheat	1 biscuit	(25 g)	3
Special K	1 cup	(250 mL)	1
Wheat bran	3 tbsp.	(50 mL)	11
White bread	1 slice	(30 g)	1
Whole wheat bread	1 slice	(30 g)	2

To ensure adequate fiber in the diet it is only necessary to restrict the intake of refined cereals and sugar and eat a preponderance of whole-grain cereals, fruits, and vegetables. If your family is accustomed to white bread, soft drinks and other refined carbohydrate products, this may be easier said than done. If you can't switch them to whole-grain bread you can at least add three tablespoons (50 mL) of wheat bran to their breakfast cereal every morning. You can also have raw fruits and vegetables always ready for snacks.

Sometimes we don't eat things simply because they aren't easily available. One of our children gave a teenage party one night and provided all the usual potato chips, cheesies, soft drinks, and cake. She also prepared a large tray of carrot and green pepper sticks, cauliflower stalks, cherry tomatoes, and celery, figuring it would look pretty for the party and her own family would eat it the next day. She left the kids alone for a while. When she returned to check on supplies she found that there were still plenty of starches and sweets, but the vegetable platter was bare.

REMEMBER

We need carbohydrates, sugars and starches for energy—they are inexpensive and the body converts them to the blood sugar glucose.

The don't make us fat unless we eat more than we need; then the body converts them to fat and stores it.

If you have to choose between sugar and starch, you are further ahead cutting down on sugar and favoring starchy foods.

If you have developed a sweet tooth and you are hooked on sweets, try sugar substitutes in moderation while de-programming yourself away from expecting sweetness in foods.

Always make sure you eat whole-grain cereals and bread as well as plenty of fruits and vegetables; they contain fiber, which is an undigestible form of carbohydrate. It facilitates the bowel movement and may help protect against cancer of the colon and heart disease. If you are a white bread eater, add three tablespoonsful of wheat bran to your cereal every morning.

Chapter 6

Calorie-Maker
Number Three: Proteins

How much in a weiner? Several years ago Ralph Nader sailed through our town knocking everyone flat with fear. His pronouncement? Hot dogs contain only 12 per cent protein!

What did this mean to a nation of weiner eaters? Was it much too little? How much harm does a 12 per cent hot dog do? The panic eventually subsided and we are now able to place the weiner in perspective. From a nutritional point of view we should calculate protein as a proportion of the calories, rather than of the weight, in the food. In weiners, 16 per cent of the calories are protein. The real reason for concern is not that hot dogs contain 16 per cent protein calories, but that they contain 80 per cent fat calories.

The protein content of a hot dog is actually quite respectable. There is no such thing as a 100 per cent protein food. All protein sources contain large amounts of fats, carbohydrates, and water and probably quite a bit less protein than you have been led to believe. People on so-called high protein diets are advised to eat steak and cheddar cheese, for example. The proportion of calories from protein in round or T-bone steak is at most 50 per cent (and 50 per cent fat), cheddar cheese is 25 per cent protein and 75 per cent fat, while fillet of sole is almost 80 per cent protein (with 20 per cent fat). While all these foods are rich in protein, they (except for the sole) are even richer in fat. They contain no carbohydrates.

There are rich sources of protein that contain no fat, but are high in carbohydrates. Take, for example, skim milk, with 40 per cent of calories from protein and 60 per cent from carbohydrates; cooked red kidney beans with 25 per cent protein calories and 70 per cent carbohydrate calories; whole wheat bread with 16 per cent protein and almost 80 per cent carbohydrate calories; and oatmeal porridge with 15 per cent protein and 70 per cent carbohydrate calories. This is why we need to eat a variety of sources of protein to ensure the right balance of fat and carbohydrates. Remember, we want our diets to have no less than 10 per cent of the calories from protein, no more than 30 per cent from fat and the remaining 60 per cent from carbohydrates.

There are plenty of high protein foods listed in the NutriScore chart. You will find them in areas A, B, and G. If you score well in these areas, you will be getting plenty of protein; more, in fact, than you need.

What is protein used for? Protein is necessary for the constant building and rebuilding of every cell in our bodies. It and other nutrients are used in the performance of the various functions of the body. Proteins produce enzymes that cause life-sustaining reactions in the body. There are enzymes to handle every nutrient in our food. For example, there are enzymes called amylases in the mouth and intestines that convert the starch in our foods to the sugar maltase. The enzyme maltase in the intestine converts it to glucose (blood sugar) which passes through the intestine wall into the blood to be distributed to various tissues such as muscle, brain, and liver. In every cell of these tissues there are about thirty enzymes involved in breaking down glucose to give the cell the energy it contains; about four calories for each gram of glucose. Without these enzymes, the body can't use the food it receives.

We must have amino acids to make protein. Amino acids look like beads, and proteins are like long bead chains twisted together. The body breaks down the protein it receives from foods into amino acids, reorganizes them, and then forms its own protein. Of about twenty amino acids in all protein foods, only nine cannot be formed or transformed by our bodies and must be in the diet in the right amounts. These are called essential amino acids and are listed among the nutrients in Chapter 7. The other amino acids in protein (sometimes referred to as nonessential) can be transformed in the body and therefore are not needed in precise amounts, but we should have a good supply of them.

For high nutritional value, protein should contain the essential amino acids in the amounts needed by our bodies, plus a generous quantity of the nonessential amino acids. Animal proteins such as milk, cheese, eggs, meat, chicken, turkey, and fish are all high-quality proteins.

Low nutritional value proteins usually have one or more essential amino acids in short supply. They are found in plant products such as bread, buns, spaghetti, macaroni, breakfast cereals, beans, peanuts and peanut butter, and soybeans.

We can get high nutritional value proteins by combining foods. For example, the cereal proteins in bread, buns, spaghetti, macaroni and breakfast cereals are of low quality, mainly because they contain very little of the essential amino acid lysine. Lysine is in plentiful quantity in legume proteins, as in beans, peanuts and soybeans. So, if we combine a cereal-protein food like bread with a legume-protein food like peanut butter we produce a food of high nutritional quality: the peanut butter sandwich.

Mixing animal and cereal proteins also results in high quality nutrition. A sandwich of cheese, meat, fish, chicken, turkey or eggs provides many essential and nonessential amino acids. Most breakfast cereals, *when taken with generous quantities of milk*, provide high nutritional quality protein. And the economical, ecologically sensible practice of mixing extruded soy protein with hamburger meat is perfectly safe, because the soy-hamburger mix offers just as high quality protein as hamburger meat alone.

The vegetable plate. Vegetarianism, whatever its ideological basis, only makes sense nutritionally when a combination of foods is used to provide high quality protein and other nutrients.

There are many types of vegetarians, ranging from those who eliminate meat but allow eggs and milk (the most common type) to those who eliminate meat and eggs or meat and milk, or all three.

Adults, and only adults, can safely remove meat, but nothing more, from their diets. The more animal products we eliminate, the more difficult it is to balance the diet nutritionally. Given our present knowledge of nutrition, it is possible for adults to eliminate meat, provided that eggs and milk and their products are included in the diet and dishes with high quality protein combinations of cereals and legumes are substituted for the missing meat. Many nutritionally sound meals can be devised by using cereals such as bread and rice and such legumes as broad beans, chick peas, lentils, soybeans, and kidney beans.

Children and adolescents up to the age of twenty should not have any group of food eliminated from their diets. While we believe that adults should never be permissive at the table and should definitely prohibit non-nourishing foods, we also believe that to remove a whole group of foods from a young person's diet is unfair and risky. Occasionally, an allergy to milk or eggs or shellfish will make that particular food undesirable, but to eliminate the entire animal protein source at the very time the body has an enormous need of first-quality protein for growth is to ask for trouble.

Women of child-bearing age on a vegetarian diet should think beyond protein. They should be aware that their iron needs are great.

With the use of enriched or whole-grain bread and cereals the amount of iron may be pretty well maintained without meat, but women in these years might find an iron supplement necessary and should check with their physicians.

Vegetarians should also be aware that meat, particularly liver, contains vitamin B_{12}, which cannot be found in cereals and legumes. A vitamin B_{12} supplement may be necessary.

Of course, once a woman becomes pregnant, she is feeding an embryo, and vegetarianism becomes risky for the fetal growth. We therefore do not recommend such dietary restrictions during pregnancy or while nursing a baby.

The quality of protein in grains and cereals is particularly important to a vegetarian. The quality is higher in whole-grain bread and cereals than in refined products. All cereals contain limited amounts of lysine, and it is the lack of lysine that makes them low-quality protein. Most of the lysine is in the germ. When the germ is removed, very little lysine remains in the refined product, and the protein value of the cereal drops even further.

Baking has virtually no negative effect on the quality of bread protein, except possibly in the crusty part of the loaf. On the other hand, processing can lower the protein quality of breakfast cereals substantially. Puffing, for example, requires heating the cereal at very high temperatures under high pressure. This often destroys some of the lysine and lowers the nutritional quality of the cereal protein.

Sugar-coating once again can spell disaster. The sugar-coating can result in immobilizing lysine so that it cannot act with other amino acids, and separately the amino acids are of no use. All or nothing is the principle governing their effectiveness. Why do we have to sugar-coat a perfectly good cereal? Just to program our taste buds to expect every food to be sweet.

Two advantages to vegetarian meals deserve mention. One is that a properly balanced vegetable plate can reduce the amount of fat in our diet while maintaining the quantity and quality of protein. Ths other is that animal protein may be conserved and the more easily produced plant substances may be utilized. It takes seven to 20 pounds or kilograms of plant protein to produce one pound or kilogram of meat protein: that is, a steer must eat seven to 20 times as much grass, legume, or cereal protein for every unit of weight of animal protein its body provides. A cow must eat five pounds or kilograms of plant protein for every pound or kilogram of milk or cheese protein we hope to get from it. Clearly it saves both land and money to eat the plant protein ourselves.

Although we can't eat grass, we certainly could eat legumes and cereals. Soy protein has been used for animal feeding in North America for many years. Recently, advanced technology has enabled us to extrude, or spin, soy proteins into simulated meat form, and we now have soy sausages, bacon bits, and ham slices. Soy could also be converted into curd to simulate milk or cheese. If there is the predicted land crunch in future years we can expect to see a lot more soy simulated foods.

Proteins are involved in some allergies. It may be hard for those of us who do not come from allergic families to credit an allergy to such basic, everyday food as milk or eggs, but it does happen. Allergies may be related to various substances in foods, but one frequent cause is the absorption of undigested protein. When a food protein enters the bloodstream, the immune system in the body reacts violently, producing allergy signs.

Normally when we eat protein the digestive system breaks it down into amino acids and only these are absorbed by the intestine and turned into body protein. Any protein not made in the body is not normally allowed into the bloodstream. However, in some people a malfunction of the absorption system does allow undigested protein to enter the bloodstream. The body then reacts in the same way it does to infection or to a tissue transplant. The immune system goes into play and tries to protect us by annihilating the foreign matter.

If a person tends to absorb a particular protein, he may well absorb that protein wherever it is found. Thus if you absorb milk protein without digesting it, and hence display allergic reactions whenever you drink milk, you are also likely to respond adversely to yogurt, cheese, ice cream, and many other products containing milk proteins.

Reading labels becomes a way of life for allergic individuals. Eating out can be a traumatic experience, because the waiter or waitress may not know exactly what is in a dish, and may be unable to find out. The listing of ingredients, particularly on institutional-size containers of commercial products, is so vague and incomplete that it is often of little value to the allergic individual. When dining out, stick to simple foods such as tomato juice (not soup), steak, broiled fish, bread and fruit for dessert.

Liver is such a valuable protein food that if we had to advocate only one meat food, it would be liver. It is particularly rich in protein and also contains iron and most vitamins and minerals.

It is only recently that we are recognizing the nutritional value of liver and the demand for it is increasing. And consequently, we are paying highly for it, particularly for calf and baby beef liver. But, pork and chicken livers are still inexpensive. They offer the same nutritional value as beef liver, which makes them a real steal.

REMEMBER

To balance your diet, at least 10 per cent of your calories will have to come from protein. How can you be sure? Score well in areas, A, B, and G of NutriScore.

You not only need protein, but you need a high-quality protein by combining cereal protein with that of milk, cheese, meat, egg, or peanut as in breakfast cereals with milk and in cheese and other sandwiches.

Yes, you can become a vegetarian and remove meat from your diet, but only if you know enough about nutrition and if you are not a child or a teenager (their nutritional needs are so high that vegetarianism becomes too risky). We also don't recommend vegetarianism for pregnant women or nursing mothers.

What Makes Our Bodies Tick?

Chapter 7

We Are a Bundle of Chemicals, and Wet One at That....

Nourishing our bodies is no easy matter. The process demands that we supply all the chemicals that our bodies cannot make for themselves. There are fifty of these chemicals and among them are vitamins, amino acids (which make proteins), fatty acids (which make fat), minerals, water, and oxygen. And here they are: the "fabulous fifty!"

Water
Oxygen
Amino Acids in
Proteins
Lysine
Methionine
Threonine
Tryptophane
Leucine
Isoleucine
Phenylalanine
Histidine
Valine
Fatty Acids
in Fats
Linoleate
Linolineate
Arachidonate
Carbohydrates
Glucose
(may be formed
from starches
and sugars and
certain amino
acids)
Fiber

Vitamins
Vitamin A
Thiamin (B_1)
Riboflavin (B_2)
Niacin (B_3)
Pyridoxine (B_6)
Pantothenate
Biotin
Folate
Cyanocobalamin (B_{12})
Ascorbate (C)
Calciferol (D)
Tocopherol (E)
Menadione (K)
Minerals
Calcium
Phosphorus
Iron
Sodium
Potassium
Chlorine
Fluorine
Iodine
Sulphur
Magnesium
Manganese

Copper	Selenium
Cobalt	Vanadium
Chromium	Nickel
Molybdenum	Silicon
Zinc	Tin

The perfect diet contains all these nutrients in the amounts needed by your body. NutriScore helps you achieve this balance in your diet. Follow it and score up to the levels specified for your age in each area of the chart. As you go through this book and pick up more nutrition information and use it every day, you will get closer to eating a perfect diet.

The most plentiful nutrient is water. Even when drinking milk or juice, we are drinking mainly water. Milk is 88 per cent water and so is orange juice. We *eat* water, as well. Hard cheese is 40 per cent water, cottage cheese 80 per cent, cucumber and watermelon are 95 per cent water. When we're hungry the extra nutrients in these water-logged foods and drinks are beneficial, but if the problem is thirst, the cheapest, simplest, most satisfying solution is to turn on the tap and pour ourselves a long, cold drink.

We need water first and foremost. The fasting feats of Ghandi, the Vietnam protestors, Dick Gregory, the Irish nationalists and the many other passive resistors of our time all are based on the deprivation of food, not water. To make their demonstrations effective the fasters must remain alive, and they can do this on little or no food, but without water they would soon die.

Water is the main component of the body, accounting for two-thirds of its weight. Without water, nutrients and other necessary substances could not be transported to the cells, tissues and organs where they are required. Blood is mainly water, and the whole circulating system with its arteries, aortas, lymphs, and capillaries is a magnificent waterway along which nourishment is carried to its destination and waste is collected for excretion. Excretion itself requires water for the formation of stool and urine.

Dehydration doesn't happen normally because each of us comes equipped with a thirst-regulating mechanism in the brain that tells us when our bodies need water. We automatically feel thirsty and drink. There are stories of people surviving on life rafts by drinking urine, but even this wouldn't keep them alive for long because each time the urine passed through the body it would both pick up further pollutants and diminish in quantity. The body requires a constant supply of fresh water to function, and your chances of surviving are a lot better if you're lost on a snowy mountain peak (like the Andes, where melted snow kept plane crash victims alive) than if you're lost in a desert or marooned on the ocean. You can't see dehydration at work. You don't shrivel like a prune when you get dehydrated nor plump up like a soaked raisin when you drink. When dehydration is in its advanced stages you don't even feel thirsty.

A hangover is your body complaining that it's been robbed of water. Alcohol is a great dehydrator. For every ounce or milliliter of alcohol we drink, the body uses eight ounces or milliliters of water in its disposal. If you drink four ounces (118 mL) of scotch on the rocks within an hour, your body has to come up with a quick quart of water (almost 1 L) to handle the alcohol. If you space out the drinks the strain on the body will be less. You still might get the dry mouth, the queasy tummy and the headache if you take more alcohol, or take it faster than your body can handle, but if you learn your limit and keep in mind that alcohol demands extra fluid which has to come from your body, the morning after shouldn't be so bad. It's colorful but incorrect to refer to an alcoholic as an "old soak" and speak of "drying him out"; actually the large quantity of liquor he consumes has already dried him out.

Having a cold is like being lost in the desert. We need fluids to get through it. Consider the extra water we need for coughing, sneezing and making the mucous that fills our sinus. And if all of this doesn't dry you up, a fever surely will. Perspiration is our way of cooling the feverish body. We need extra fluids to compensate for this loss.

Your baby may lack water, too. Once, on a four-hour transcontinental flight, a baby in the next row started crying. His mother had finished feeding him about an hour earlier. We weren't changing altitudes, the air pressure was constant. The mother responded rather reluctantly, asking for another bottle of formula. The airline hostess suggested water for the baby. She knew her business; the air on a plane is dry and often makes a baby thirsty. The mother refused. The baby took only a little of the formula and a little while later he was at it again, screaming his head off. The airline hostess returned, this time with a bottle of water. She said, in a rather firm but compassionate tone, "I have a baby of my own and I know how thirsty they can get." It worked; the baby gulped the water down. So, the next time your baby frets between feedings, think thirst first.

REMEMBER

Your body needs 50 chemicals for its nourishment. NutriScore was designed to give you all of these in the right amounts. Using the information in this book plus the scoring system will bring you closer to eating a perfect diet.

Of all the nutrients you need, water is the most plentiful. Your body comes equipped with a fine regulating mechanism that makes you feel thirsty when the water needs of the body are not met.

You may still get in a state of dehydration when you drink too much (alcohol, that is) or when you have certain infections such as a cold. Babies often get thirsty when mothers forget to give them a bottle of water once in a while.

Chapter 8

What Makes Our Bodies Tick?
Vitamins—The Bs and C

Vitamins are the best known of all nutrients, thanks to the near-miraculous improvement in our health resulting from their discovery early in the twentieth century. Nutrition became a publicly recognized science when young mothers, themselves bowlegged from childhood rickets, found they could protect their children from the disease by simply ensuring that they received sufficient vitamin D. As they watched the baby's legs grow strong and straight their belief in the power of vitamins strengthened as well.

Unfortunately, public understanding did not keep pace with public admiration for the new pills, and soon people began "pill-popping," acting on the principle that if some were good, more was better. This misconception of our need for vitamins persists today and has given rise to the various "mega-vitamin" theories and therapies and to ortho-molecular medicine. A sane look at vitamins will show that we need them in small, but (and this is the important point) constant quantities.

Vitamins help in various biochemical reactions. The vitamins themselves do not participate, but they assist in body reactions such as those freeing energy from carbohydrates, fat, and protein; those forming the immune system; and those which detoxify some of the poisonous substances entering the body with food and drink and air. Most of the vitamins work as helpers to enzymes.

Only small amounts of any vitamin are necessary or safe. Minute amounts of a vitamin are all that are required to help in the body reactions. When you take very large quantities of a vitamin pill, sometimes the body's reactions are forced to an unusually high level. If for any reason you drop your vitamin pill for a day or more and your body returns to normal levels, the body will feel deprived and respond as if it had a vitamin deficiency. Of course, if the body tended to store an excess of a vitamin, taking and storing too much of it would be simply poisonous in the long run. For the vitamins that the body doesn't store, the extra amounts go out in the urine and this can be hard on your kidneys. For these reasons it is dangerous to follow the unproven theories about mega-vitamins and ortho-molecular medicine and take more than the normal requirement of vitamins. Never take two if one will do.

Taking too many vitamin pills is unbalancing our diets. Many people feel a false sense of security because they take vitamins regularly. They look upon this as insurance against malnutrition. This may be the case, but it doesn't mean that they can go ahead and eat or not eat anything they want. Nothing could be further from the truth.

A "vitamin supplement" should contain what is missing from the diet. We now pick vitamin pills to contain as many ingredients and as much of them as possible, but we overlook that we should first find out what we are missing.

Before you take vitamins, score your diet to find out what is missing. Use the NutriScore rating system. If your score is low in areas E and F you should be thinking of folic acid and vitamin A. If it is area C that has the low score, vitamin C is the one you should be concerned about. And if you score low in areas A, B, and G, you should pay more attention to the B vitamins. NutriScore helps balance your diet and ensures the vitamins you need.

The choice is yours: food or pills. The amount you need of each vitamin could be obtained by eating more of the food shown in the appropriate area of the rating chart to raise your score. Or, you may consult the amounts suggested for vitamins and mineral supplements in the following table. These are based on recommended intakes in the United States, Canada, and the United Kingdom (Appendices B, C, and D). As with foods, a vitamin and mineral supplement should be carefully selected. Choose one to give you no more than your daily needs at the lowest price available. Just remember that if you take a vitamin C pill, you are getting vitamin C alone, but if you eat an orange you get not only vitamin C but many, many other nutrients in amounts that would help balance our diet.

Your guide to how much of each vitamin and mineral you should expect in a supplement—not too much and not too little.

THE B VITAMINS

The B vitamins are often promoted by health food proponents in the form of yeast tablets or dessicated liver. These sources can vary in their content of the B vitamins depending on the method of preparation, and

If the supplement (pill, chewable tablet or syrup) contains:	The amount in a daily dose should not be less than:	need not be more than:
Vitamins:		
Thiamin (B_1)	1.0 mg	5.0 mg
Riboflavin (B_2)	1.0 mg	5.0 mg
Niacin	10.0 mg	50.0 mg
Pantothenic acid	50.0 mcg	200.0 mcg
Pyridoxine (B_6)	1.0 mg	5.0 mg
Biotin	2.0 mg	10.0 mg
Folic acid	100.0 mcg	400.0 mcg
Vitamin B_{12}	2.0 mcg	6.0 mcg
Vitamin C	30.0 mg	200.0 mg
Vitamin A	2,000 iu	10,000 iu
Vitamin D	200 iu	400 iu
Vitamin E	10 iu	100 iu
Minerals:		
Calcium	0.1 g	1.0 g
Phosphorus	0.1 g	1.0 g
Potassium	0.1 g	1.0 g
Magnesium	0.1 g	0.5 g
Iron	5.0 mg	40.0 mg
Copper	0.5 mg	3.0 mg
Manganese	0.5 mg	5.0 mg
Zinc	5.0 mg	25.0 mg
Iodine	50.0 mcg	300.0 mcg

it is not desirable to take yeast tablets on a regular basis as they tend to be gas-forming, which can cause discomfort.

Thiamin (vitamin B_1) is needed for the metabolism of carbohydrates, and the more carbohydrates we eat, the more thiamin we need.

Thiamin is found in many foods: pork cuts, beef cuts, liver of any animal (calf, pork, or chicken), and in whole grain or enriched bread or cereal. These foods are in areas A and G of the rating chart. Since thiamin is not stored in the body to any great extent, and is readily excreted in the urine, it is essential to include thiamin in your diet everyday.

The symptoms of thiamin deficiency include at first loss of appetite, constipation and digestive disturbances. There will be depression and irritability as well as inability to concentrate or take an interest in work. More advanced symptoms include numbness or prickliness in the toes or feet. The ankles may become stiff and lose their reflexes. In the later stages of the deficiency, various nerves and muscles will be affected and the heart function will be disturbed.

Alcoholics are the most likely candidates for thiamin deficiency because alcohol interferes with the absorption of several B vitamins, including thiamin.

Riboflavin (vitamin B$_2$) is needed for the metabolism of proteins. It is related to the amount of protein in the body or what nutritionists call the lean body mass or, in simple terms, the muscle mass.

Riboflavin is found primarily in milk. In addition, it is obtained from liver, kidney and heart and also enriched cereals and bread. These foods represent those listed in areas A, B, and G of the rating chart.

Ribovflavin is constantly excreted in the urine. However, there are indications that some of it is stored to a limited extent in the liver and kidney. This may be because it is tied up in its action to protein which is also stored to a very limited extent in the liver and the kidney.

A shortage of riboflavin in the diet shows as reddening and swelling of the lips and the tongue, inflammation and cracks in the corner of the mouth and at the nasal angles, burning and itching sensations in the eye and scaliness of the skin, particularly in skin-folds around the joints. But, weather conditions, particularly severely dry and cold atmospheres, could also cause reddening and swelling of the lips and the inflammation of the corners of the mouth, and anyone who reads and writes most of the day may well get burning and itching sensations in the eye. So, do not be convinced by symptoms alone. Riboflavin deficiency is not likely to develop unless you have a general deficiency of protein and other B vitamins.

You should be concerned about riboflavin deficiency if you do not habitually include in your diet such foods as milk, yogurt, cheese, liver, kidney or heart, and if you depend mainly on starchy foods. Teenagers and adults who follow restrictive bizarre diets are also in danger of developing riboflavin deficiency.

The Zen Macrobiotic diet contributes to riboflavin deficiency. The diet progresses through seven levels becoming more and more restrictive. The most advanced level is limited to brown rice only. At this stage the protein intake and that of several vitamins, including riboflavin, is sufficiently low as to cause a state of deficiency.

Exposure of milk to sunlight lowers the amount of riboflavin because riboflavin is sensitive to light. This is a problem when milk is packed in transparent glass bottles and delivered outside homes in full exposure to sunlight. North Americans remember amber milk bottles for home delivery. These were designed to eliminate riboflavin loss. Nowadays, cartons and plastic jugs have solved the problem.

Niacin (or nicotinic acid or vitamin B$_3$, B$_5$, or G) is involved in the release of energy from carbohydrates, fats, or proteins. It acts in close association with thiamin and riboflavin. Because of these complex interrelationships the need for niacin is dependent on the caloric consumption. The higher the caloric intake, the greater the need for niacin. It is also closely related to protein intake in that one of the amino acids in protein—i.e., tryptophan—is converted to the body to niacin and foods that are high in protein provide the body with a source of niacin.

The main sources of niacin in the diet are meat, legumes, or pulses such as peanuts, beans and peas, and whole-grain or enriched cereals or bread. These represent the foods in areas A and G in the rating chart.

Niacin deficiency symptoms are neither specific nor clear-cut because niacin is involved in the metabolism of carbohydrate, fat, and protein and could be formed from one of the amino acids in protein. Historically, niacin has been recognized as the pellagra prevention (P-P) factor. Pellagra is a disease characterized by weakness, lassitude, loss of appetite, and eruption of darkened scaly dermatitis in skin areas that are exposed to the sun. It was common in populations that depended on corn as the staple item in the diet, as in the southern part of the United States. Now, a case of pellagra is simply unheard of. It is a disease that belongs in the archives of medicine as far as the United States and Canada are concerned.

Niacin will neither cure nor prevent schizophrenia. It has been tried as therapy for schizophrenia but has proven to be of no use in either prevention or cure of the disease. Evidently, assuming a connection between the symptoms of niacin deficiency and of schizophrenia, two doctors, Abram Hoffer and Humphry Osmond, used massive doses of niacin to treat schizophrenic patients back in 1954. They claimed dramatic cures, and in the years that followed, various researchers in the field of psychiatry and mental health tried massive doses of niacin for therapy, but to no avail. At least one large study that was approved beforehand by Dr. Hoffer showed niacin ineffectual in curing or even alleviating the symptoms of schizophrenia. To date, much of the testimonial evidence in support of the use of niacin in treating schizophrenia is hard to accept.

Pantothenic acid is needed for the metabolism of carbohydrates, fats, and proteins. It is involved in the synthesis of cholesterol, steroid hormones, and hemoglobin (the substance containing iron in red blood cells).

Pantothenic acid is found in meat, chicken, milk, eggs, peanuts, beans, peas, broccoli, kale, sweet potatoes, yellow corn, and whole-grain cereals and bread. This represents the foods in all areas, except area H, of the rating chart. The friendly bacteria living in our intestines make large quantities of pantothenic acid, which our bodies absorb and use all the time. The intestinal bacteria make an unknown quantity, and the total intake must satisfy our nutritional needs, for we have never observed naturally occurring deficiency signs in humans. This is why nutrition scientists have been unable to determine how much of this vitamin our bodies need. It is estimated that the North American diet contains about 10 to 20 mg of pantothenic acid a day.

Pantothenic acid will not restore color to gray hair, contrary to what Adelle Davis said. In several experiments, volunteers took antagonists (chemicals that block the action of the vitamin in the body) to develop deficiency symptoms. They suffered from fatigue, headache, sleep disturbances, nausea, numbness, muscle cramps, and tingling of the hands and feet. One symptom that appears in deficient rats, but not in humans, is the graying of hair. The addition of pantothenic acid to our diets does not reverse the graying of our hair. However, Adelle Davis claimed that it does and suggested that all gray hair is a symptom of multiple nutritional deficiencies of para-aminobenzoic acid (which is not even a vitamin), biotin, folic acid, and pantothenic acid. She declared, "I have seen many people whose hair returned *temporarily* to its natural color after they had followed adequate diets especially rich in all the B vitamins." (Emphasis is ours.) We recommend very strongly that you, the reader, follow an adequate diet especially rich in all the B vitamins but do not be disappointed if your hair remains gray, because you will feel younger than the color of your hair suggests.

Pyridoxine (vitamine B$_6$) is needed for the metabolism of proteins, including absorption of amino acids in the intestines and their transport from tissue to tissue in the body. Pyridoxine is also involved in the formation of niacin from the amino acid, tryptophan. Our body's need for pyridoxine depends on the amount of protein we eat; the more protein we consume, the more pyridoxine we need.

The foods that can claim to be rich sources of pyridoxine are limited to whole-grain cereals or bread, liver, kidney, and various meat cuts. These are the foods represented in areas A and G of the rating chart.

Pyridoxine deficiency can occur, as was cruelly demonstrated in the United States in 1951. Canned reconstituted baby formulas were introduced on the market as a convenience to the mother who did not wish to take the time to reconstitute the powdered formulas. Soon babies across the United States who were fed the liquid formulas began showing such scary symptoms as irritability, muscular twitchings, and convulsions. Babies on similar formulas sold in dry, powdered form did not show these symptoms.

The convulsing babies owed their lives to the alertness of nutrition scientists at the Food and Drug Administration who related these symptoms to the convulsive seizures in pyridoxine-deficient rats. A supplement of the vitamin corrected the situation and cured these babies promptly. Apparently the liquid formula had to be sterilized in the can. This heat treatment was sufficient to destroy the pyridoxine in these formulas and deprive the babies of the vitamin. It wasn't hard to correct this anomaly by adding more of the vitamin to the liquid formulas so that even with the great loss during sterilization enough was left to satisfy the nutritional needs of the babies.

In addition to the convulsive seizures displayed by the liquid formula babies, pyridoxine deficiency causes greasy dermatitis around the eyes and at the corners of the mouth. Prolonged deficiency of the vitamin in the diet could lead to dizziness, nausea, vomiting, anemia, and kidney stones.

If antagonists tie up the action sites of pyridoxine in the body, deficiency symptoms can develop even when the diet contains adequate supplies of the vitamin. In the case of pyridoxine, one such antagonist is a chemical called isonicotinic acid hydrazide (INH) which is used for the treatment and prevention of tuberculosis. The dangers from INH are real in northern communities, where Inuit are often given a constant supply of the drug. Physicians in the North who administer INH without giving an adequate pyridoxine supplement (50 to 100 mg of the vitamin are needed daily) could be subjecting the population to the dangers of pyridoxine deficiency.

Oral contraceptives increase the need for pyridoxine. These hormones create a physiological condition in the body similar to pregnancy which raises the need for several vitamins, particularly pyridoxine and folic acid. In fact it has been demonstrated that a supplement of 50 mg of pyridoxine daily eliminates many of the side effects of the contraceptive pill, including mental depression.

Biotin is involved in the metabolism of fat and protein. Biotin is found in many foods, especially egg yolk, liver, and kidney. The average North American diet provides 0.2 to 0.3 mg of biotin a day. In addition, bacteria in our intestine make biotin and we absorb most of it. So, it is difficult to know how much biotin our bodies get every day. This makes it hard to determine how much we need.

About the only time we face the chance of being deficient in biotin is when we eat raw egg white. This doesn't happen often but there are those who are fond of egg nogs or Spanish Smiles in plentiful supply. Actually, you'd need to consume about eight or ten raw eggs to be affected and the cholesterol and saturated fat that you get from eating that many eggs should discourage you at the outset.

In any case, we seldom eat raw egg white alone. In egg nogs, we mix milk and eggs. In Spanish Smiles, it is egg, milk and orange juice. And we always use whole eggs. Egg yolk is rich in biotin but raw egg white contains a protein called avidin, which ties up biotin in the intestines and prevents it from getting into the blood stream. However, heating, even slightly, destroys avidin's ability to tie up biotin; so commercial egg nog, which has been pasteurized, does not tie up biotin and does not bring about deficiency symptoms.

The symptoms of biotin deficiency are exzema of face and body, hair loss, and paralysis. In the unhappy event that you ever develop such symptoms, don't jump to the conclusion that you are deficient unless you have been eating raw egg whites.

Folic acid (folacin) is needed for the metabolism of proteins and nucleic acids. The nucleic acids are substances formed by each cell for the reproductive process and the transfer of hereditary characteristics from one generation of cells to another as the body grows.

Folic acid is widely distributed in green vegetables; its name is derived from "foliage," or leaf. Since folic acid is easily destroyed in cooking, it is important to eat fresh green vegetables or ones cooked very little in small amounts of water. Storage of fresh leafy vegetables for several days at room temperature without refrigeration can cause substantial loss of folic acid. Animals store large quantities of the vitamin in the liver and the kidney, and these two meats from any animal (beef, veal, pork, or chicken) are considered rich folic acid sources. Even the cooking of liver and kidney destroys very little folic acid. These foods are found in areas A and E of the rating chart.

Folic acid deficiency is possible because of the limited number of foods considered rich in folic acid. Anyone who does not eat fresh green vegetables or liver or kidney regularly should worry about the possibility of being deficient. You don't have to eat them every day, since your body stores the vitamin in the liver and kidney and uses it as needed.

The main sign of folic acid deficiency becomes evident upon medical examination of the blood. The condition is known as macrocytic anemia. The red blood cells are enlarged and there aren't as many of them as in healthy blood. They also contain less hemoglobin, the red pigment with iron in it that carries oxygen around the body.

Other signs of folic acid deficiency include smooth red tongue, gastro-intestinal disturbances, and diarrhea.

Studies in the United States and Canada, as well as in other countries, revealed that many people of all ages and of both sexes do have lower than normal levels of folic acid in the bloodstream. This suggests that many of us are eating diets that are low in folic acid. The best thing to do for your own protection is to eat a green vegetable once a day and liver or kidney once a week. It would do you more good than relying on a vitamin pill, because the leafy vegetables and the liver or kidney would give you many other vitamins, as well as minerals and protein.

Vitamin B_{12} (cobolamin) is needed for the metabolism of proteins and nucleic acids as well as that of fat and carbohydrate. The vitamin's function is so closely related to protein metabolism that the vitamin B_{12} requirement increases with the increased consumption of protein. B_{12} is also involved in the formation of red blood cells and the prevention of pernicious anemia. In this role, it is associated with folic acid. This is the reason that when the intake of folic acid is high (from vitamin pills) there is a danger of masking some of the pernicious anemia symptoms. It seems sensible, therefore, that in formulating a vitamin pill, folic acid and vitamin B_{12} be together and in the amounts needed in the body.

Pernicious anemia can only be diagnosed medically. It may develop in some individuals even when the diet is adequate in B_{12} and folic acid. In these individuals, who are rare, there is a special protein lacking in the intestine. This protein is needed to carry vitamin B_{12} from the intestine to the blood stream. Its absence is an inherited condition. The only treatment is frequent injections of vitamin B_{12} to avoid dependence on the intestinal route to get the vitamin into the blood stream.

Sources of vitamin B_{12} are foods of animal origin. Plant products do not contain vitamin B_{12}. Even yeast, which is regarded as a good source of other B vitamins, is not a source of B_{12}. The richest sources are liver and kidney of any animal (beef, lamb, pork, or chicken) because these animals store the vitamin in the liver and kidney. We humans do, too. Other good sources of B_{12} are meat, fish, eggs and milk. This presents a problem for strict vegetarians who restrict their diets to plant products even to the exclusion of eggs and milk. In planning a vegetarian diet, it is important to only restrict meat. Even then, it would be of definite benefit to allow liver and kidney once a week. Under no condition should such restrictions be imposed on children's or adolescents' diets. The growing years require protein and all the vitamins and minerals needed for its metabolism, of which vitamin B_{12} is one.

In simple dietary deficiency of vitamin B_{12}, symptoms develop that range from sore tongue, back pain, weakness, loss of weight and a prickly sensation in the extremities. In prolonged deficiency of the vitamin, mental and nervous defects develop and lead to death. Of course, dietary deficiency could be avoided by eating the right foods.

VITAMIN C

Vitamin C (ascorbic acid) is needed for the metabolism of proteins and many amino acids. It is also important to the absorption of iron from the intestine and to the storage of iron in the liver.

It is needed for the normal function of the adrenal glands. The concentration of vitamin C in these glands is particularly high. These glands secrete into the blood stream the hormone adrenaline or epinephrine which helps the body cope with stress conditions such as shock, anxiety, and injury. This does not mean that the body needs "more than usual" amounts of vitamin C to cope with normal everyday stress. The body builds its defenses by storing the needed vitamin C in the adrenal glands all the time. Large intakes of vitamin C do not help you cope with stress better. But, with proper eating habits which fulfill your body needs of vitamin C and other nutrients regularly, your defense mechanism against stress will be there when you need it. Our needs for vitamin C are set at 30 to 60 mg a day.

Vitamin C is in many fruits and vegetables. It should not usually be necessary to supplement the vitamin C in a balanced diet because even the high level of 60 mg is contained in four ounces (75 mL) of orange juice, a medium-sized orange, a medium-sized grapefruit, four ounces (12 g or about ten) of fresh or frozen strawberries, half a medium-sized cantaloupe or a half cup (125 mL) of cooked and drained broccoli or brussels sprouts. In addition, green leafy vegetables and peppers are rich in vitamin C and are often combined in fresh green salads. Other fruits and vegetables rich in vitamin C are listed in area C on the rating chart.

Potatoes could be an important source of vitamin C if eaten when freshly dug, boiled or baked, and in large quantities (one medium-sized potato would contain 20 mg of vitamin C). The amount of vitamin C drops to a third after six months of storage. Extensive processing, as in producing instant dehydrated potatoes, potato chips, or preheated frozen french fries, reduces the amount of vitamin C drastically.

In areas of the world where fresh fruits and vegetables are not abundant and potatoes are consumed in large quantities, potatoes contribute most of the vitamin C in the diet. Such was the case in

England. The introduction of instant dehydrated potatoes on the British market in the late 1950s presented a serious hazard to health, since much of the vitamin C was destroyed in the processing. This brought about an outcry from nutritionists which led to the enrichment of dehydrated potato granules with vitamin C.

Several exotic fruits and other sources of vitamin C, such as rose hips, are promoted by health food stores. These are often expensive sources, are not as available nor as esthetically desirable in our diets as the many fruits and vegetables rich in vitamin C. These exotic products are promoted as "natural sources" of high vitamin C potency, competing with vitamin C pills, made from "synthetic" vitamin. We are not against rose hips. If you grow roses, you may wish to harvest the base of the rose flowers after they ripen into a red or orange color in the fall and use them in making jam. Use them but don't rely on them for your vitamin C. They are not your everyday dish.

Vitamin C deficiency results in many signs of tissue damage, particularly the connective tissue that holds skin, muscles, tendons, and bones together. This shows up in the form of bleeding gums, delayed healing of burns and wounds. Another sign of tissue damage resulting from vitamin C deficiency is the tendency of small blood vessels under the skin to hemorrhage, creating many tiny red spots.

Vitamin C and the common cold. The evidence for needing vitamin C in the event of a cold or any other infection cannot be denied. Under such conditions, the body loses more than the usual amounts of vitamin C. The need for the vitamin is increased, but *not* to a level one thousand times that normally needed by the body.

Proponents, such as Linus Pauling, of high intakes of vitamin C for the prevention and cure of the common cold recommend taking a gram, that is 1000 mg, of the vitamin every day to prevent colds and 4 to 6 g per day to cure them. It is clear that such amounts could not normally be supplied in natural foods.

There is no scientific reason for taking such large quantities of vitamin C. Vitamin C is an acid and as it gets excreted in the urine, it turns the urine to acid. This causes many salts to be excreted, which could be a strain on the kidney function. Also, there is evidence that the body adjusts to the high intakes to the point that if you miss taking the vitamin C tablet and your intake drops to around normal levels of, say, 30 to 60 mg, deficiency signs develop.

The scientific evidence available for the argument for increased amounts of vitamin C to prevent and cure the common cold falls on major studies conducted at the University of Minnesota in 1951 and at the University of Toronto in 1974. In both these double-blind studies, half the volunteers received vitamin C tablets, while the other half, unbeknown to them or to the researchers, received placebos (a dummy tablet that looks, tastes, and smells like a vitamin C tablet but doesn't have any vitamin in it). Only after the experiments were over was the code deciphered and those who received the vitamin tablets were distinguished from those who got the placebo. These studies showed that intakes as high as 1 g of vitamin C per day do not prevent a cold. Those getting the vitamin tablets had as many colds as those on dummy tablets.

However, those getting as little as 20 mg vitamin C (in the Minnesota study) or as high as 4000 mg vitamin C (in the University of Toronto study) during their colds, suffered for about one-third less time than those receiving normal intakes of vitamin C. A repeat study at the University of Toronto reported in 1975 did not show any value for the high intakes of vitamin C.

It is quite possible that vitamin C intakes of 200 mg a day during a cold would help cure it sooner. But other measures would help cure the cold as well. Do not overlook resting in bed and taking plenty of fluids. The body loses a lot of fluid in the form of mucous during a cold. It is important to compensate the body for the water lost. Drinking orange juice (freshly squeezed, canned, or reconstituted frozen) or eating oranges would meet the body's need for water and vitamins pleasantly and healthfully. Instead of one small glass of orange juice (about 60 mg vitamin C) every day, try four of them, one every four hours. That will give you as much as 240 mg vitamin C, about 15 ounces (450 mL) of water, and many vitamins that will contribute to your body's nourishment.

If your cold is not severe enough to keep you in bed and you cannot be close to oranges and orange juice, try a 50 mg vitamin C tablet four times a day and drink water or other nonalcoholic beverages often. You may have difficulty finding vitamin C tablets of lower potency than 100 mg each. In this case, split each into two and take only half a tablet at a time.

It is preferable to space vitamin C supplements over the day since it is excreted in the urine shortly after consumption. It fact, in some nutrition courses, students checking for vitamin C in urine collected during the four or six hours after a high vitamin C supplement find they recover almost all the supplement within that period. It goes through the body so fast that it can present a strain on the kidneys if taken regularly in excessive amounts.

Cigarette smokers lose more vitamin C from their bodies than do nonsmokers. However, we do not know how much, if any more vitamin C, smokers should take in their diet to compensate for the loss. It would be safe, however, to suggest that heavy smokers no more than double their regular intake of 30 to 60 mg. But then, heavy smokers should be trying to quit smoking altogether. Taking more orange juice or fresh tossed salad is not going to prevent lung cancer or heart disease that smokers invariable court with each cigarette.

Some people don't get enough vitamin C either from food or pills. It may seem unreal in a society where people are debating the need for gram quantities of vitamin C that some are not getting the required amount. Nutrition surveys in the U.S.A., Canada, and England found many on marginal or lower than adequate intakes of the vitamin. So we can see both extremes, those who are swallowing pills and loading their bodies beyond capacity and those who are not getting enough.

If you want a vitamin C supplement, be sensible. Buy the lowest concentration at the lowest price possible. There is no difference between the "synthetic" vitamin C and the "natural" sources. Anyone needing vitamin C will respond in exactly the same way to a tablet made with the "synthetic" vitamin as to one made with a natural "rose hip extract." In fact if you don't need more than 200 mg (and you won't), why not rely on oranges or grapefruit or their juices or other fruits and vegetables? They will supply not only vitamin C but a large assortment of vitamins and minerals that will contribute to your nutrition, health, and vitality.

REMEMBER

You don't burn vitamins for energy. Therefore, the amounts you need are small—so small, in fact, that you can put them all in a little tablet or capsule. This presents a danger. If you are pill-popping happy, you can hurt yourself.

It is safer to rely on foods, not pills for your vitamins.

NutriScore will tell you what you may be missing: area E gives foods with folic acid, areas A, B, and G for the other B vitamins, and area C for vitamin C or ascorbic acid.

The B vitamins do a lot for you. Thiamin or B_1 helps you use carbohydrates. Riboflavin (or B_2) and pyridoxine (or B_6) and folic acid and vitamin B_{12} help you use proteins. Biotin helps you use fats and proteins. Niacin or B_3 and pantothenic acid help you use the calories in food. They are all important.

Vitamin C helps you use proteins and absorb and store iron. It may also reduce the severity of colds (it doesn't prevent them).

The golden rule is to remember that the body benefits from the right amount of vitamins and not from the massive doses that some faddist suggest.

Chapter 9

Vitamins A, D, E and K
Make Us Tick, too . . .

The only reason we separated vitamins A, D, E and K from the B vitamins and vitamin C is that these are stored more readily in the body. You should be extremely careful not to take supplements with more than the suggested dosage (see table in Chapter 8.)

As with other nutrients, focus your attention on NutriScore to balance your vitamins. You will find vitamin A foods in areas B, E, F, and those enriched with vitamin D in area B. Vitamin E comes from the whole grains in area G, and vitamin K will be supplied by foods in areas A and E.

VITAMIN A

The most important function of vitamin A (retinol) in the body is in forming and keeping healthy the epithelial tissue, which is the shield the body forms to protect it from infections and other external hazards. Skin is epithelial tissue; so are the mucous linings of the mouth, the stomach and the intestines (small and large), and the mucous linings in the respiratory, genital and urinary tracts.

Rich sources of vitamin A include liver, kidney, fish liver oil, eggs, whole milk, and yellow and green vegetables (carrots, sweet potatoes, squash, spinach, broccoli) and some fruits. Eating liver and kidney once a week, eggs three times a week and vegetables and fruits daily should give us all the vitamin A we need. To rate your diet for vitamin A, watch your score in areas B, E, and F in the rating chart.

The major source of vitamin A in our diets is yellow and green vegetables. In these foods, vitamin A is in the form of carotene. Our bodies have the capacity to convert carotene to vitamin A in the intestines and in the liver. However, we always have very small amounts of carotene circulating in the blood. This does not seem to have much value since the body uses only vitamin A.

Carotenes are usually yellow, orange, or reddish in color. In some vegetables, this color is masked by the green of chlorophyll. Not every green vegetable contains carotenes. Remember the ones that do contain carotenes include spinach, broccoli, and kale.

There are many carotenes and they vary in their nutritional quality. Some are converted to vitamin A more efficiently than others. Beta-carotene is the most efficiently converted form and therefore it has the highest nutritional value of all the carotenes. However, this form is seldom found alone. Most yellow and green vegetables contain a mixture of carotenes. The intensity of the color, yellow or green, is usually a reliable measure of the content of carotenes or vitamin A.

A deficiency of vitamin A causes the skin and the mucous linings to become dry, flat, and scaly. This invites infections and allows germs to penetrate into the body. Our resistance to infectious diseases of all kinds is very much dependent on having enough vitamin A and a healthy epithelial tissue. So our parents were very wise in insisting on a spoonful of cod liver oil with breakfast during the winter months, when green and yellow vegetables weren't plentiful.

We shouldn't forget, either, that the epithelial tissue around the eye cavity dries up in vitamin A deficiency. In its advanced stage, this leads to a disease, xerophthalmia (pronounced zer-of-thalmia), in which the tear secretion stops, eyelids swell and become sticky (as bacteria infects them and fills them with puss) and eventually bacterial infection of the eye causes ulcerations on the cornea and blindness.

This condition is common in many countries where vitamin A is lacking in the diet. One estimate put the number of children going blind each year because of vitamin A deficiency at 80 000, with about half of them dying of this deficiency.

In North America, the evidence for vitamin A deficiency, while not alarming, should be of concern. We should be concerned that recent surveys found many Canadian and American children have low concentrations of the vitamin in the blood. Analysis of livers of adult accident victims in the U.S. and Canada showed many to have below average or low concentrations of vitamin A. This is an indication of a long-term deficiency state.

Recent studies also showed that the absence of vitamin A increases the susceptibility of the epithelial tissue not only to infections but also to carcinogens. This opens a new vista that suggests vitamin A protects the body from carcinogenic substances. For example, researchers at the Massachusetts Institute of Technology have shown that rats deficient in vitamin A develop more colon tumors (cancerous growth in the epithelial tissue of the colon) caused by the carcinogen aflatoxin. The same study showed rats on normal intakes of vitamin A resisted the carcinogen successfully. Remember normal intakes will do it. There is no need for excessive intake.

Similar results were obtained by researchers at Oak Ridge National Laboratory. Rats receiving adequate levels of vitamin A resisted the effect of the carcinogen methylcholanthrene and developed fewer lung tumors (cancerous growth in the epthelial tissue of the lung) than did those not receiving vitamin A. Again it should be clear that while vitamin A deficiency may increase our susceptibility to carcinogens, excessive intakes of vitamin A do not offer any more protection or allow us to consume more carcinogen. At levels higher than the recommended dosage of vitamin tablets, vitamin A could be equally as deadly as carcinogens.

The chances are that moderate long-term deficiency of vitamin A affects some of us. This will not lead to blindness, but it may well lower our resistance to disease and infections, and it can be avoided easily through sensible eating.

Sometimes parents feel desperate about their children's dislike of liver, kidney, fruits and vegetables and they give them vitamin A and D in cod liver capsules. If you feel you must do this, be careful to measure out the capsules in small dosages, every other day or twice a week. Such capsules should be kept out of reach like any drugs and poisons. In the meantime, work to introduce sound eating habits in your children by setting an example and choosing the right foods. It is the best investment for the health and happiness of your children.

It is very important not to exceed the safety limit in taking vitamin A supplements. Vitamin A (unlike the B vitamins or vitamin C) is fat soluble and therefore circulates very little in the blood stream and is not excreted in the urine. Most of the vitamin not immediately used by the body is stored in the liver. This means that high intakes of the vitamin from tablets result in large stores in the liver. If in excess, these could be toxic and lead to serious illness and death. This is why the Food and Drug Laws in Canada and the United States now do not allow more than 10 000 units of vitamin A in any vitamin tablet. The requirement in the diet is half this much, about 5000 units per day. The dangerous level is 50 000 units, which is in only five tablets.

Toxicity from over-consumption of vitamin A has been reported in Arctic explorers who have eaten the livers of polar bears, seals, Greenland foxes, and Eskimo huskies. These animals store unusually large quantities of the vitamin in their livers. There have also been reports in medical literature of children accidentally poisoned by taking large doses of vitamin capsules that were left within their reach. In addition, there have been several reports of adolescents and adults taking large amounts of the vitamin to cure a number of diseases ranging from asthma to acne to sensitivity to sunlight, thereby developing acute symptoms of toxicity.

A physician in Trail, B.C., Canada reported the case of a girl, aged 15, who took 200 000 units of vitamin A daily to treat acne. She bought tablets of 50 000 units each at the local drugstore but was advised to ignore the one-tablet-a-day dosage declared on the label as "it was quite common to take more than this in the treatment of acne." She did not lose her acne. What is more, she developed severe headaches, vomiting, and double vision along with high spinal fluid pressure. She made a complete and dramatic recovery by simply discontinuing the vitamin A tablets.

Vitamin A will not improve your sight, but a deficiency can make it worse. Vitamin A has gained the reputation over the years as the vitamin that will make you see in the dark. Children have been told if they eat carrots, they will be able to see in the dark. This is not quite true. The truth is that a vitamin A deficient individual may detect difficulty in adjusting from strong light to darkness or vice versa. When you leave a darkened theater in the middle of an afternoon performance and go into the bright sunshine you feel blinded for about a minute. Anyone would feel blinded for a second; that is natural. It is when the blinding effect is prolonged that you should become concerned.

Contrary to what many of us might have heard about the magic effects of vitamin A, it does not cure color blindness. This impression originated when scientists found that vitamin A forms part of a pigment in the retina which influences color vision and seeing in bright light. But the scientific evidence is clear that when a person becomes deficient in vitamin A, color vision is not altered but the ability to see in bright light is affected.

VITAMIN D

Vitamin D (calciferol) is essential for forming bone and keeping it strong. Bone is made from calcium and phosphorus, and vitamin D helps the absorption and utilization of calcium and phosphorus.

Vitamin D is formed by the action of sunlight on 7-dehydro-cholesterol (part of the oily lubricating substance in the skin). This is why vitamin D is sometimes referred to as the "sunlight vitamin." The cholesterol derivative is a necessary part of the formation of vitamin D, which explains why, although excessive cholesterol can be very threatening to our health, we do require small amounts.

Recent studies have shown that the skin has a controlling mechanism that prevents the formation of too much vitamin D. In countries with plenty of sunshine, as in Africa, the skin of the natives darkens into a deep tan, which slows down the formation of vitamin D. In countries with little sunshine and where the climate is too cold to encourage exposure to sunlight, as in northern Europe and America, the capacity of the skin to form vitamin D is high.

Except for the vitamin D added to milk, food contains very little vitamin D. It is as if nature intended us to get our supply from exposure to sunlight. Foods of plant origin, like cereals, vegetables and fruits, contain no vitamin D. Animal foods contain small amounts, particularly in liver where it is stored, and in fatty fish, eggs, and milk. It is a common practice in many parts of North American and some European countries to enrich milk with vitamin D. This usually ensures adequate supply among milk drinkers. However, those who do not drink milk or are not exposed to sufficient sunlight would have a limited supply.

The deficiency of vitamin D shows as rickets in children and as osteomalacia in adults. Rickets in children is characterized by poor calcification of bones, particularly long bones. The classical bowed legs are an obvious sign that may mean rickets. This has to be verified by X-rays for there are other conditions that make the legs bow. Another sign is called rachitic rosary, which is the development of bead-like protrusions on the ribs. If discovered early, rickets can be treated with vitamin D and adequate intake of milk. But it has to be diagnosed and supervised by a physician. Otherwise, bone deformities may stay with the person for life.

Osteomalacia is the loss of calcium from the bones. It may develop in mothers who do not drink much milk and do not get enough vitamin D, following a series of pregnancies and lactations. The symptoms include pain and tenderness in the bones and pressure in the pelvis and lower back and legs. One danger of osteomalacia is the slow healing of any fractures because the bones lack the ability to deposit calcium in the absence of the needed amount of calcium and vitamin D.

The amount of vitamin D in human milk is small, usually about 20 units per day which is far short of the recommended level of 400 units. This means that breast-fed babies will have either to receive a supplement (vitamin drops) or be exposed to sunlight. In warm weather, the baby may be placed naked in the warm sun rays. The baby's sun baths can begin with short periods, about three to five minutes, and increase gradually to 20 or 30 minutes. Watch carefully for skin sensitivity.

In many areas of North America and Europe, exposure to sunlight is limited and the use of ultra-violet or sunlamps is impractical. None of these methods can be relied on to meet the body's vitamin D needs. So we have to ensure that the vitamin is added to foods or included in vitamin tablets. In this lies a danger of over-consumption.

Vitamin D is toxic when taken at concentrations only four or five times the levels recommended. This is not likely to happen from foods. Rather, it results from zealous swallowing of too many vitamin D pills. There have been cases of children being poisoned by swallowing too many vitamin D pills. Initially they lose their appetites, become excessively thirsty, vomit, lose weight, and become irritable. They also have high levels of calcium in the blood and deposit calcium in the kidneys and the lungs. This condition, if allowed to go on, can result in death.

There have been cases of excessive intake of vitamin D in adults, particularly in old people suffering from loss of bone calcium. Some physicians treat this condition with massive doses of calcium and vitamin D. The patients become depressed and psychotic, lose their appetites, become excessively thirsty, and sometimes complain of weakness in the legs and difficulty in walking. Response to stopping the vitamin D is usually dramatic, with improvement in both the mental and the physical state of the patient.

Use extreme caution when taking a vitamin supplement that contains vitamin D (or vitamin A, E, or K; they are all fat soluble and therefore stored in the body). Some faddists, which unfortunately include a few physicians, promote high intakes of the vitamin for the treatment of a variety of diseases ranging from asthma to arthritis. If you have a friend or a doctor who tries to talk you into this, ignore their advice. You'll be glad you did.

Our need for vitamin D is not great. North American adults can fulfill their vitamin D requirements with half a pint (300 mL) of milk (to which vitamin D is added at the dairy) per day. Children need the amount of vitamin D contained in a quart (1.25 L) of milk. (The amount of vitamin D to be added was based on the amount of milk a child should drink in any case, and vitamin D was added because it would then be coupled with calcium.)

VITAMIN E

Vitamin E is the most talked about vitamin. To some people, vitamin E is a household word, a miracle drug that cures diabetes, arthritis, ulcers, warts, infertility, acne, coronary heart disease, and cancer.

Some athletes speak of possessing extraordinary powers and physical ability when they take vitamin E supplements. And, amidst these startling claims, nutrition scientists concede that vitamin E is needed for health but (and here follows the *truth* about E!): excessive amounts of the vitamin do not cure all these diseases, will not make you sexier than you really are, and will not make you Olympic material.

Why vitamin E is needed is not clear, except that it gets oxidized much more easily than most other substances in the body. This way it protects important substances, like vitamin A, from being oxidized and destroyed. Vitamin E is also known to protect cell membranes from highly oxidizing substances called peroxides which occur naturally in the body.

The important sources of vitamin E include salad oils, shortening and margarine, whole-grain cereals, wheat germ, liver, beans, and most fresh green leafy vegetables. In North America, possibly one half of the vitamin E in the diet comes from oils, margarine, and shortening, and the other half from all other foods combined.

Vitamin E deficiency symptoms are mainly of hematological nature. The membrane of the red blood cells becomes fragile and ruptures readily when exposed to oxidizing agents. As a result a premature destruction of the red blood cells can occur. In animals, other symptoms of vitamin E deficiency have been observed, including paralysis and muscle degeneration.

There have been a few deficiency cases reported. The most dramatic case was that of eleven premature infants who were on a synthetic formula, with insufficient amounts of vitamin E. As a result, they developed hemolytic anemia (a condition of premature destruction of red blood cells). In addition, there have been deficiency cases reported in Uganda and Egypt. In controlled experiments on men volunteers in Illinois, however, the deficient diet was fed for three years before symptoms developed. Possibly their body stores of the vitamins were sufficient to carry them for that long.

How much vitamin E we need depends on age, sex, and what kind of fat we eat. If the fat in the diet is highly saturated (butter, cheese, shortening, regular margarine, coffee whiteners with coconut oil, untrimmed steaks, eggs, etc.) you will need less vitamin E than if you eat a lot of polyunsaturated oils (safflower, soybean, corn and cottonseed oils, soft margarine and nuts). An adult man eating an average North American diet should have 10 to 15 mg or units (they are the same) of vitamin E every day. The average intake in the United States and possibly also in Canada is about 10 to 20 units per day. Recent studies in Britain showed the majority of diets tested to contain less than 10 units per day. So, the amount of vitamin E in our diet is marginal, and we should know what foods supply it and eat more of them.

Do we need vitamin E pills? Certainly not if you eat whole-grain cereals and breads, have about two tablespoons (25 mL) of wheat germ a day, eat green salads and use oils on your salad and in cooking. Often, when we say that, the question comes back, rather persistently, "But, if I don't, how much vitamin E should I take?" Our answer is, "If you must take a vitamin pill, then make sure you don't take more than 15 units of vitamin E a day at the most." Well, have you tried buying a vitamin E pill with 15 units in it? They don't make them that way. Usually, they start at 100 units per capsule and go up from there. And, these are capsules that you can't split six ways to get 15 units. The answer is simple; take a capsule of 100 units once a week. Since the body stores vitamin E you won't lose it and the body will use the weekly supply just as well.

Because it is fat soluble, the blood (which is basically water) cannot carry much of it and the kidney doesn't get rid of it, so the body has to store what is not used. It is held in fatty tissue like the adipose tissue (under the skin, around the belly) and the sex glands like the ovaries and the testes. If the intake is too high the accumulation of vitamin E may well interfere with the function of these tissues and glands.

Why do so many people think they need vitamin E pills? They are influenced by the promotion talk of the manufacturers of the vitamin, and the faddists who back them, wittingly or unwittingly. The two main conditions for which massive doses of vitamin E are promoted are: improved athletic performance and treatment or prevention of coronary heart disease. In either case, the proponents of vitamin E claim that while diets may be adequate to prevent vitamin E deficiency, supplements are needed for extraordinary athletic performance and for a strong heart beat.

Only physical training (and not vitamin E) will improve athletic performance. This was proved in a recent study reported from Britain. The researchers used two matched groups of boys, similar in age, weight and physical ability. One group received 400 units of vitamin E every day and the other had none (except what was in their food). For six weeks, both groups underwent intensive physical training. Before and after the six weeks, they were subjected to tests of physical ability and endurance including pull-ups, push-ups, sit-ups, running and swimming performances. The six weeks of physical training improved their ability and endurance capacity just as well whether they had the vitamin E therapy or not.

Vitamin E will not cure or prevent coronary heart disease. The erroneous idea of treating coronary heart disease with massive doses of vitamin E has been an embarrassment and worry to the medical profession for years. In the late 1940s, Drs. Evan Shute, Wilfred E. Shute (brothers) and Albert Vogelsang (all of London, Ontario) reported great success in the treatment of angina pectoris (chest pain associated with coronary heart disease) with vitamin E. This aroused medical interest all over the world. Vitamin E therapy was tried and failed in the treatment of angina pectoris patients in many medical centres, including Mount Sinai Hospital in New York, the University of Manchester in England, and Duke University in North Carolina. Nonetheless, the Shute brothers continued to claim success for vitamin E in the treatment of various forms of heart disease. And, the manufacturers of the vitamin, particularly through health food stores, capitalized on this medical claim. As a result, many vitamin E enthusiasts promote the vitamin for anyone who hopes to prevent a heart attack. And, here lies the danger: not only is vitamin E of no value in treating heart disease, but for anyone suspecting a heart condition, delaying a visit to the physician could be fatal.

Did we say you should have 10 to 20 units a day? We did, and here's where to find them:

> in 2 tbsp. (25 mL) wheat germ
> in 4 slices whole-grain bread
> in a bowl of green salad with oil as dressing, plus oil used for
> broiling and frying.

An effective measure to increase one's intake of vitamin E would be increased consumption of whole-grain cereals and wheat germ since this doesn't mean increasing your fat consumption.

Two tablespoonfuls (25 mL) of wheat germ a day would adequately supply each of us with the vitamin E we need. It can be sprinkled on hot or cold cereals or used as an ingredient in pancakes, muffins, breads, or loaves.

Wheat germ is a delicious coating for panbroiled or baked fish, especially if you add some chopped almonds for additional texture, and an attractive topping for baked meat loaf and all your favorite casseroles. Broil or pan fry with safflower, sunflower, soy, corn, or cottonseed oil, and the vitamin E is increased yet again.

And a final word to the economy-minded. Don't throw away the wilted green leaves of vegetables. Dark green, leafy vegetables contribute a good amount of vitamin E, even more if they are wilted! So cast a second glance at the outside leaves before you toss them away. Cooked quickly or eaten in a salad, they are better sources of vitamin E than the crisp inside leaves we treasure.

Try a wilted spinach salad with orange slices, lettuce, and garlic dressing with finely chopped egg white and capers.

Use the outer leaves of cabbage for cole slaw. If they're beyond serving as a salad, slice into bite size, and add them to vegetable soup during the last 15 minutes of cooking.

When someone advises that you look to vitamin E as a rejuvenator and aid for your mid-life doldrums, don't search at the drug counter! Smile and serve them wheat germ pancakes and waffles, wheat germ scallopine (toss 6 tbsp. (100 mL) in with the crumbs), green salads, and whole-grain cereals and breads. And relax, while you enjoy the taste: delicate, nutty and filled with health-giving nutrients served up with loving care!

Wheat germ—raw or toasted? Raw wheat germ, because it contains oil, can go rancid. Chances are, if you ever taste wheat germ which has gone "off" slightly, you will never want to eat it again. So buy it fresh and always refrigerate it. The toasted wheat germ which costs so much more than raw is processed to stop the chance of rancidity and allows you to keep it at room temperature.

If you prefer the flavor of toasted wheat germ, toast the raw wheat germ yourself by baking it, spread on a baking sheet at 200°F (100°C) until it toasts to a golden color. It has a more nutty flavor like this and adds to the taste of foods when you serve it as a sprinkler (desserts and cold cereals).

VITAMIN K

Vitamin K is the coagulation vitamin. It is needed for the natural process of blood clotting. In case of injury or internal hemorrhage certain proteins coagulate to form a clot that prevents further blood loss. These proteins are formed in the liver with the help of vitamin K, then released into the blood.

Foods which are considered rich in vitamin K include all green leafy vegetables, egg, soybean oil and liver. The amount needed by an adult is estimated to be about 30 mcg, which is very small and easily supplied to the North American diet. The vitamin is stable to cooking and oxidation.

In the case of a deficiency, blood clots will be slow in forming or may not form at all, thus endangering the life of the person.

This type of hemorrhage is quite different from that in hemophilia, a hereditary disease which does not respond to vitamin K. Hemophilia is caused by the inheritance of a defective chromosome. If the newborn is a boy, he will be hemophiliac; if a girl, she will be a carrier and could pass it on to her children. The disease became famous when it was discovered that Queen Victoria was a carrier of this disease which plagued European royalty for three generations. Even now, the prospect of it reappearing among her male descendants is of real concern.

Giving anticoagulants has been the only way to produce vitamin K deficiency. In some circulatory disorders, such as the phlebitis that hit President Nixon in 1974, blood clots readily in the blood stream and threatens to block the flow of blood, which could lead to death. In these cases, anticoagulants are given to counteract the action of vitamin K and prevent the formation of clots.

There is danger in taking excessive vitamin K only when taking it in vitamin tablets. The form of vitamin often used in these tablets has been found to be toxic when taken in excess. This is why our food and drug regulations control the form and the amount of the vitamin in supplements and in food.

REMEMBER

Your body stores more of vitamins A, D, E and K than it does of the Bs and C. Be careful that you don't take too much or you may just, literally poison yourself.

It is safer to get these vitamins from food. You will find the vitamin A foods in areas B, E and F and those enriched with vitamin D in area B. Vitamin E is in whole grains in area G and vitamin K foods are in areas A and E.

You need vitamin A for healthy skin and mucous tissue. If deficient, your skin and mucous would dry up and make you susceptible to infections.

Vitamin D is necessary for healthy bones. If you are a child, a vitamin D deficiency could mean a case of rickets. If you are a grownup, it may weaken your bones and slow the healing of any fractures.

Vitamin E protects tissues and cell membranes against oxidation. You need it but not in massive doses. But it wouldn't cure or prevent a heart attack, turn you into an athlete or make you sexier.

Vitamin K protects you from bleeding to death if you are injured. It helps the natural process of blood clotting.

Chapter 10

The Salt of the Earth—Minerals

You are the salt of the earth. That's no flattering metaphor, it's the literal truth. Our bodies contain the same minerals as the earth; in fact, they contain minerals *from* the earth, passed on to us via our food. When we eat adequate servings of plants grown in mineral-rich soil, and of milk, eggs, and meat from birds and animals fed a diet suitably high in minerals, we obtain all the minerals needed by the human body.

Our bodies use minerals to build the structural skeleton and to help enzymes in life-sustaining reactions.

The bulk of the body minerals are in the bones, which are mainly calcium and phosphorus, plus small amounts of other minerals including magnesium and fluoride. The soft tissues also contain a full range of minerals in small quantities. The body of a 160-pound (75 kg) man would contain about 5 pounds (22.5 kg) of minerals, of which about 2 pounds (900 g) are calcium and approximately one pound is phosphorus. In addition, there are 4 ounces (120 g) of potassium, 2 ounces (60 g) of each of sodium and chlorine, about half an ounce (15 g) of magnesium and one-tenth of an ounce (3 g) of iron. Fourteen more minerals are present in such minute quantities that they have come to be known as trace minerals.

We need minerals the way we need vitamins, in small but constant supply. Many vitamin pills contain a few minerals, particularly iron. Our selection of a supplement should be based on the amounts suggested in Chapter 8. Find out what you need and buy the best value. Under no condition should such a supplement substitute for food. Most minerals can only be obtained from foods.

Again, NutriScore ensures a wide variety of minerals to meet your body's needs. The foods in area A are particularly important for their iron, magnesium, and zinc content. Those in area B have calcium and phosphorus. Foods in areas C, D, E, F, and G provide a wide range of minerals, particularly trace minerals, the combination of which could not be matched by any tablet or capsule on the market today.

PHOSPHORUS

Most of the phosphorus our bodies require goes to form bones and teeth. The remaining body phosphorus (about 20 per cent) is in soft tissues. Every cell of the body contains phosphorus. It forms part of nucleic acids which are needed for protein formation and for the transfer of hereditary characteristics from one generation of cells to another: it is part of the phospholipids which help move fats around the body; and it is needed for the metabolism of carbohydrates and the release of energy from them.

Phosphorus is in practically every food. There is really no problem getting enough phosphorus in our diets. Foods rich in phosphorus include meat, fish, poultry, eggs, cheese, milk, nuts, legumes, and whole-grain cereals and bread. In addition, the liberal use of phosphates as preservatives in processed foods contributes further substantial amounts.

A superfluity of phosphorus, not a deficiency, is likely to be the problem. If the diet has too much or too little phosphorus in relation to calcium our bodies will not use calcium efficiently. We make the best use of calcium in our diet when it contains one or two parts phosphorus to one part calcium. In North America it is unlikely that the phosphorus will be less than that range. Recent evidence suggests that phosphorus is exceeding the desirable level with increased consumption of meat (rich in phosphorus) and with the widespread use of phosphates in processed foods. The outcome is an increase in our bodies' needs for calcium which might become difficult to satisfy.

CALCIUM

Calcium is used first and foremost to form our bones and teeth. Ninety-nine per cent of the calcium in the body is in the bones. The other one per cent, however, is hard at work in the blood and other fluids and in soft tissues. In the blood, calcium works hand-in-hand with vitamin K to ensure blood clotting when needed. In tissues, calcium helps healthy muscle tone and nerve function. We maintain in our bodies a very delicate balance between calcium on the one hand, and sodium, potassium and magnesium on the other. This balance is necessary for normal rhythmic contraction and relaxation of the heart muscles. Our bodies recognize the need for calcium in such crucial tasks and readily take it from bones whenever it is needed in the blood or elsewhere in the body.

Among the foods that are excellent sources of calcium are milk, hard cheeses (like cheddar), dark green leafy vegetables and fish with soft bones (like salmon and sardines). These are followed by legumes (like beans), soft cheeses, eggs, and nuts.

Calcium deficiency in early life can seriously inhibit the growth of bones and teeth. The need for adequate supply of calcium (and phosphorus) starts early in the formation of the fetus. It gets them from its mother's blood and bone. It is crucial, therefore, that the pregnant woman receive adequate amounts of calcium and phosphorus. If the supply is not sufficient during pregnancy and later on in infancy and early childhood, one of three things may happen: (1) the offspring may not grow, or (2) the bones and teeth become malformed as in rickets with bowed legs and protruding ribs, or (3) the bones and teeth developed may be of poor quality which means more fractures and slow healing capacity in later years. Thus one could have a full-sized skeleton (i.e. grow tall) but have brittle bones, delicate and undermineralized. The bone deformation in rickets may be due to lack of vitamin D, or of phosphorus, as well as too little calcium.

Lack of calcium or phosphorus during pregnancy influences the development of teeth and jaws. It may result in narrow face and jaws and overcrammed teeth in a narrow dental arch, which may well affect the looks of the child. Such deficiencies during the formative years may be difficult to correct later in life.

If the calcium shortage continues throughout life, the bones gradually become demineralized and develop into a condition known as osteoporosis. The bones become porous, thin, and fragile. As a consequence, they are susceptible to fractures that are slow in healing. This condition is fairly common among our senior citizens. While some respond to calcium therapy, it is often difficult to correct the effects of years of low intake of calcium. The insult to the body is so severe that it is beyond repair.

Three factors affect the utilization of calcium by the body. The first, as we have already mentioned, is the amount of phosphorus in the body in relation to the amount of calcium. The balance should be one of two parts of phosphorus to one part of calcium.

The second factor is the amount of protein in the diet. Excessive intakes of protein result in lower calcium absorption. Foods that are rich in protein, but have little calcium, should be consumed in moderation and combined with rich sources of calcium. Again, meat is such a food (plenty of protein, plenty of phosphorus, but little calcium). To balance the effect of meat, milk, cheese, and beans (all are good sources of protein and calcium) should be included in the diet. Meat should always be eaten in moderation. We do not need very much of it, but we don't need to drop it from our diets completely. Our servings need not exceed 3 or 4 ounces (85 to 115 g) rather than the overwhelming 16-ounce (450 g) steak.

The third factor that affects the utilization of calcium is vitamin D. It is necessary for calcium absorption in the intestines. In its absence, rickets develop even though calcium in the diet may be adequate.

Do you, or your children, lack calcium? You can get an idea of how adequate the calcium is in your diet from the score you get in area B of the rating chart. If your score is not up to par, consider the food listed on that page and the scoring factor of each. Then increase the one you like most and can afford till you score right.

IRON

We need iron to fight that tired feeling. Actually we need more than iron. We need good nourishment and exercise. But without iron, oxygen wouldn't reach the muscle to release the energy that the muscle needs to work. It is no wonder that those deprived of iron feel tired all the time. Iron has the ability to both pick up and release oxygen. It is a component of hemoglobin, which in turn is a component of the red blood cells. With the help of the iron in its hemoglobin, the blood is able to pick up oxygen in the lungs and carry it to capillaries throughout the body, where it releases the oxygen to the cells. The oxygen is then used by the respiratory enzymes to oxidize glycogen, fatty acids, and amino acids in order to release energy for the use of the muscle cells.

Good sources of iron include meat, heart, liver, shellfish, beans, peas, spinach, dates, dried fruits, nuts, eggs, whole grain or enriched bread and cereals. But getting enough iron in our diet requires careful planning, particularly for infants. They depend greatly on milk. Remember how we sometimes speak of milk as "the most *nearly* perfect food." The reason for the word "nearly" is that milk is low in iron. An infant of a well-nourished mother should have enough iron stores to last about three or four months. This is why pediatricians recommend supplementary foods (i.e., cereals and egg yolk) or iron supplements to be given at three months of age.

A deficiency of iron means that the body cannot manufacture normal amounts of hemoglobin; the size of the red blood cells will therefore be reduced and as a result the blood will transport less oxygen. With less oxygen reaching the body cells, including the muscle cells, we become weakened and feel tired and "washed out." This condition is referred to as iron-deficiency anemia.

Of course, a sedentary person with a poor circulatory system will have a slow feed of blood supply to muscle cells and to lungs. The same condition might result from the lack of physical fitness. Low hemoglobin could also result from the deficiency of copper, pyridoxine, folic acid, vitamin B_{12} E, or C. All these deficiencies are known to cause anemia in some form. Of all these, iron is the least efficiently absorbed by the body. This means that we'll have to build our iron stores slowly and maintain them at all times.

There is another interesting consequence to the shortage of iron in the body. Resistance to infection is lowered, presumably as the infecting bug tends to attract iron out of the host cells and in to its own, thus weakening the host cells and strengthening itself.

Our bodies do not absorb iron efficiently. And foods do not contain enough iron to make up for this inefficiency. It is necessary for us to pay attention not only to how much iron we are getting but how well it is absorbed. We have to build our iron store gradually. Actually, while the body is inefficient in picking up iron from foods or pills, it is very efficient in hanging on to what it's got. The body uses and re-uses iron with amazing efficiency. The only route through which the body may lose iron is blood loss in hemorrhages, wounds, and menstruation. The elaborate mechanism our bodies have to develop blood clots is a proof of their efficiency in conserving iron.

To help absorption, iron has to be in a chemical form that is biologically available. Generally speaking, iron in animal foods is more available than that in vegetable foods. Organic forms, as in meat and liver, are more available than those in pharmaceutical preparations. Even those vary among themselves. For example, iron sulphate or gluconate or fumarate is more available than iron pyrophosphate. The form of iron added to bread and cereals in their fortification may not be as available as the amount the label implies. So industry should be concerned not only about the amount of iron added to food but also about the form in which it is added.

Proteins are needed to carry the iron to the bone marrow where hemoglobin is made, to the cells where myoglobin and enzymes are made and to the liver and spleen where iron is stored. Therefore, a good source of protein in the diet is needed. This is why iron is poorly absorbed from foods low in protein such as potato chips and french fries when eaten alone or with gravy. This is an eating habit that some children and teenagers fall into.

There is also evidence that vitamin C helps the absorption of iron. So it is helpful to take orange juice in the morning with eggs.

Iron is needed in small amounts but it is needed. The body of a healthy adult contains less than a teaspoonful of iron. Yet, the maintenance of this amount is one of the main problems in North America and many parts of the world.

Let us take a teenage girl with poor eating habits. She skips breakfast and throughout the day relies on pop, candy, and chips and gravy to kill her hunger pains. She justifies these bizarre eating practices to herself because she is trying to keep slim and doesn't want to eat very much. She has no practical knowledge of nutrition. After all, from childhood her parents gave her the freedom to eat as she wished. And the school never cared what she ate or what she knew about what she should eat. Her iron (among other nutrients) intake is low. Her iron stores in the liver are low. She grows up, after a fashion, and becomes pregnant. Now her body needs for iron are increased to cover the needs of the baby. Her doctor will undoubtedly decide that she needs an iron supplement and prescribe a generous one. By the time her depleted iron stores get built up, it may be too late to help the baby develop normally and come into the world with enough iron in its blood. Since our former teenage girl, now mother, didn't know enough to feed herself properly, the chances are she will not know enough to feed her baby to build his or her iron (and other nutrient) stores.

The only way to break this vicious circle is through knowledge and the motivation to value yourself and your children.

To find out how well your diet rates as far as iron is concerned, work on the foods in area A of the rating chart. If you don't have a high enough score for yourself, adjust the foods and the amounts you eat to meet your iron needs.

SODIUM AND POTASSIUM

Sodium and potassium belong together. Sodium concentrates outside the body cells while potassium concentrates on the inside. They'll have to be in balance to maintain a normal flow of nerve signals and muscle contractions. If the balance in the amounts of sodium and potassium is upset, the nerve impulses and muscular contractions will be irregular, either too strong or too weak, and our nerve and muscle functions will be impaired.

Sodium and potassium also play a role in maintaining a balance between the acids and bases in our body fluids. Sodium is further needed for the absorption of various nutrients, while potassium is needed for energy release from carbohydrates, fats, and proteins.

Both sodium and potassium are in plentiful supply in our food.
Sodium is found in table salt which we add to foods. It is also present in
fruits, vegetables, and milk. Potassium-rich foods are bananas,
oranges, and tomatoes and their juices, potatoes, followed by a variety
of fruits and vegetables, meats and cereals.

The symptoms of potassium deficiency reflect its role in normal
muscle function. As a result the deficient person suffers muscular
weakness, heart muscle irregularities, as well as respiratory and
kidney failures.

As for sodium, the body tends to regulate its level carefully;
conserving it when in short supply and dumping the excess in urine
and sweat when the intake is excessive. However, habitual heavy use
of salt may upset the body's ability to regulate the level of sodium in it.
There is evidence that this may develop into a case of hypertension
(high blood pressure) with serious health complications in later years.
This raises serious concerns about the widespread addition of salt to
processed and home-prepared foods. Patients with high blood pressure, placed on a sodium-restricted diet by their doctors, can't rely on
processed foods; the manufacturer may have added salt. The main
thing to remember is always to read the label and ensure that no salt
has been added.

**Both sodium and potassium play a vital role in balancing the acids
and the bases in the blood and other body fluids.** It is essential that
these fluids be neutral, neither acidic nor basic. The body therefore
regulates with amazing precision the amounts of acid-forming minerals and base-forming minerals.

Sodium and potassium, as well as calcium, iron, magnesium, and
inorganic phosphorus, are base-forming. These balance the acid-
forming minerals, such as chlorine, sulphur and organic phosphorus,
which are in cereal grains, eggs, meat, poultry, and fish.

Consequently, a diet containing large quantities of meat (i.e. organic
phosphorus) is slightly acidic. To help neutralize its effect, fruit and
vegetables (i.e. sodium, potassium, magnesium, and inorganic phosphorus) are needed. A balanced and varied diet is necessary to help the
body maintain its neutral value. The acid-forming and base-forming
characteristics of many foods have an effective neutralizing influence
on the body which is essential because the enzyme reactions of the
body can only proceed in a neutral environment. There are just two
compartments of the body where the environment does not have to be
neutral: the stomach is acidic and the intestine is basic.

To maintain the balance between sodium and potassium is not
difficult, but we should check our habits and general situation for

possible pitfalls. Those of us who sprinkle generous amounts of salt on every dish should either sprinkle less or sprinkle potassium-containing salt substitutes. Children with frequent bouts of diarrhea could become deficient in potassium due to poor absorption and increased loss in urine. People on some diuretics, such as those "rainbow" reducing pills, lose so much potassium that they run the risk of a deficiency.

Human milk contains about one-third the concentration of sodium in cow's milk. A baby consuming 1 L of human milk (which is a reasonable amount) would get 160 mg of sodium. The same amount of cow's milk would give 500 mg. Obviously human babies don't need much sodium. It is encouraging that the manufacturers of baby food have refrained from adding salt to their products for some years now. Of course, you must be careful to buy only those commercial products that are without salt and be vigilant in your efforts to omit salt when preparing baby foods at home.

The myth that acidic foods can be counteracted by antacid preparations is just that, a myth.

Mass advertising promoted antacid preparations as the only way to neutralize stomach acidity, which plagues those of us who eat too fast. Some of these preparations are proudly advertised for their ability to neutralize 47 times their weight of acid. These are all unjustified claims. Our stomachs normally secrete a strong acid which is essential for the digestion of food. Attempts to neutralize the acid in the stomach are counteracted by the secretion of more acid. The body regulates this acidity in the normal healthy individual to help digestion.

There are many reasons for indigestion. High fat consumption, particularly of the overheated oils found in fried foods, is a common cause. Many times the reason is simply psychological stress or anxiety! It's not what you are eating, but what is eating you that causes indigestion. A wise person would do well to avoid antacid preparations unless advised by a physician for a specific condition.

MAGNESIUM

Magnesium is famous for its role in milk of magnesia and Epsom salts. Both are old standby medications with stomach-soothing, wound-healing, and laxative effects. Milk of magnesia (magnesium hydroxide) is an antacid which should never be used in excess. Epsom salt (magnesium sulfate) acts as a laxative because it draws a lot of water in the intestines. However, magnesium plays a much larger part in our bodies than merely neutralizing the acid in the stomach or flushing the contents of the intestines.

Half the magnesium in the body is in the bones and teeth. The other half is in soft tissues, helping the release of energy from glycogen, the making of proteins, the regulating of body temperature and the orderly contraction of nerves and muscles. It is an extremely important nutrient.

Magnesium is found in whole-grain bread and cereals, nuts, beans and green leafy vegetables. Here is a case where we can't advise you to rely on enriched bread or cereals. Enrichment of bread does not include adding back the magnesium lost in refining. If you can't give up the white bread, use whole-grain wheat, bran, or wheat germ breakfast cereals. Another point to remember is to eat some *fresh* green leafy vegetables as in salad greens. Cooking washes away magnesium. If you boil vegetables do not discard the water; use it for soups and stews.

Magnesium deficiency shows up as muscle weakness, irritability of nerves and muscles, including irregular beats of the heart muscle, and finally spasms and convulsions.

A magnesium deficiency may well develop in someone who relies on a restricted selection of food—i.e., without much variety—particularly if these foods are highly refined and processed. Old folks living on a "tea and white toast" diet do not get much magnesium. Deficiency symptoms have also been observed in alcoholics and patients who have been on diuretics for a long period of time.

ZINC

Zinc is used by the body in the formation of many hormones, including insulin, which regulates carbohydrate metabolism, and of many enzymes, including those controlling the transport of carbon dioxide in the blood.

Good sources of zinc are animal foods such as meat, liver, eggs and shellfish, particularly oysters. Whole-grain bread or cereals, wheat germ, wheat bran, beans, and nuts are less satisfactory sources because, in certain areas, the soil and hence the plants growing on it are deficient in zinc. Farm animals in these areas become deficient and have to be given supplements. This may well happen to those restricting their diet to plant foods. Furthermore, in certain cereal grains, beans, and nuts, even those grown on zinc-rich soils, the zinc is often in the bound form, which means much of it is not biologically available.

Zinc deficiency has been the subject of recent nutrition research. This was mainly a result of observing several deficiency cases in the Middle East. The symptoms included dwarfism, anemia, and slow healing of wounds. In animals, the deficiency of zinc in the diet during pregnancy results in deformities in the offspring somewhat similar to those in the thalidomide cases.

IODINE

Iodine forms part of the hormone thyroxine, which regulates various body functions, particularly the basal metabolic rate. The basal metabolism may be thought of as the minimum level of life processes. It is the energy the body needs just to exist—i.e., to go on living without moving.

The amount of iodine in food varies depending on the food and the area in which it is grown. Vegetables contain more iodine when grown close to a seashore than inland. Foods of marine origin (fish and seaweed) are richer in iodine than land animal foods (milk, meat, and eggs). Because of this variation in iodine content, many countries favor the addition of iodine to a food that is consumed by everyone. Thus, the iodization of salt is gaining wide acceptance. In countries like Canada, Switzerland, Colombia, and Guatemala the iodization of table salt is mandatory by law.

A deficiency in the iodine supply will prevent the thyroid gland from forming enough thyroxine to burn a normal amount of energy. If this occurs during pregnancy, the offspring will be a cretin, will not grow, becomes a dwarf, and will be mentally retarded. In adults, the most obvious sign of iodine deficiency is the enlargement of the thyroid in the neck, a condition called goiter. It is a reaction of the gland to the shortage in iodine. It grows bigger in the hope of soaking up more iodine, but to no avail. The thyroid enlargement could range from being undetectable without doctor's examination to being so embarrassingly obvious that the patient favors bulky turtleneck sweaters to hide it. Other signs of prolonged iodine deficiency include feeling cold even in warm weather, gaining weight, having extremely dry skin, and developing a husky voice.

Fat people should not be given thyroxine to burn off excess fat. Occasionally, a quack will argue that since people with high levels of thyroxine have high metabolic rates, which means they burn more calories than normal without having to exercise, therefore, the administration of extra thyroxine will reduce the fat person quickly and without effort. They neglect to mention that the fat burned this way is a small amount and that excess thyroxine upsets the balance of other hormones in the body, and causes accelerated heart action and traumatic emotional states of tension and nervousness. The fat person ends up in worse trouble than when he started.

Too much iodine produces the opposite effect from thyroxine: it depresses the action of the thyroid gland and the formation of thyroxine. In other words, if we take too much iodine (perhaps in the form of iodine-rich dried seaweed or iodide tablets), we achieve the same results a deficiency of iodine would produce. Moderation in all things is the answer.

In the United States, there are indications that iodine consumption is excessive mainly through additives such as iodates used as dough conditioners in making bread and iodofor, used as an antiseptic in dairy lines. TV dinners were found to contain unusually high levels of iodine. Presumably the same conditions exist in Canada. However, there are no indications that such excessive iodine intakes have interfered with the thyroid function of many North Americans.

FLUORIDE

The value of fluoride extends beyond the prevention of dental caries. Not only is fluoride deposited in the enamel of the teeth (to strengthen it against caries) but it is also deposited in the bones. The fluoride-containing bone crystals are longer lasting than the ones without fluoride. This is important in old age when the bone crystals begin to break down gradually, making the bones fragile and fractures difficult to heal—a condition known as osteoporosis. Recent medical reports have shown far fewer cases of osteoporosis in areas with fluoride in the water.

None of the foods consumed regularly contain much fluoride. Tea is a fair source of it. Sardines, eaten with bones, also contain some fluorides. In addition, dehydrated foods reconstituted with fluoridated water contain fluorides.

In the absence of fluoridated water supply, it might be necessary to give children fluoride tablets. But make sure they don't contain more than 1 mg in a daily dose. Avoid excesses and keep it up as a daily routine.

Using fluoride toothpaste and topical application of fluoride by dentists are no substitutes for fluoridated water. We need to ingest fluorides rather than to apply them externally to get the full value.

The addition of fluoride to the central water supply is a logical way to ensure that all citizens receive the necessary fluorides. Unfortunately, fluoride has been used as a political football in many communities. "To fluoridate or not to fluoridate" has puzzled many politicians in civic and municipal elections. The opponents of fluoridation have been fighting it on the grounds that fluorides are poisonous. An additional argument is that it violates the right of the individual to drink the water in its "natural" state.

The validity of these views must be questioned since the amount of fluoride could be regulated to produce beneficial effects without reaching poisonous levels. After all, the chlorination (chlorine is closely related to fluorine) of water has been practiced with an excellent safety record and without public furor. Chlorination is essential to destroy disease-causing germs that might be present in the water supply. And, if chlorination does not alter the "naturalness" of our drinking water, why should fluoridation be so accused?

The value of fluorides in fighting tooth decay is demonstrated by a classical study conducted in two small communities in New York. Newburgh had its water supply fluoridated to the level of one part per million (1 mg in every litre of water). Kingston's water was not fluoridated. The children who drank the fluoridated water had 65 per cent fewer cavities than the ones not getting fluorides—one cavity in the fluoride group for every three in the non-fluoride group.

This study has been repeated throughout North America with as good or better results in favor of fluoridation.

Modern techniques in fluoridation allow the safe addition of fluorides to the desired level. The cost is only a few cents per person per year.

Fluoridation of the central water supply is necessary only when the level of fluoride naturally present is below one part per million, and only to bring it up to this level.

THE TRACE MINERALS

There are many other minerals needed by the body in very small quantities. We often can't determine how much of each of these "trace" minerals we need, nor how much of them is in the various foods. The chemical and biological analysis of these trace minerals has presented technological difficulties. Nonetheless, we know that when these minerals are absent from diets, animals don't grow normally and the newborn may be deformed and become subject to a variety of diseases.

The only way we can ensure adequate supply of trace minerals is by including in our diets many unrefined wholesome foods: whole grain breads and cereals, fresh or dried fruits and raw vegetables, nuts, organ meats (liver and kidney), and shellfish. We don't need very much of these minerals but we cannot do without them.

REMEMBER

Minerals are critical for your nourishment. They are numerous but we lack information on some of them. The only way you can be sure you are receiving an adequate amount is by eating a wide variety of wholesome foods.

NutriScore helps you ensure a balance of minerals in your diet. You get iron, magnesium, and zinc from foods in area A, calcium and phosphorus from those in area B, and the wide range of other minerals from areas C, D, E, F, and G.

You need calcium and phosphorus to form bones. If you don't have them you may not grow to full size and/or your bones and teeth will be weakened.

Iron helps the body use oxygen and release energy from food. With good nourishment and exercise, iron can help you fight that old, tired feeling.

Sodium and potassium work together to help the flow of nerve signals and muscle contractions and to balance the acids and the alkalies in the body. To keep them balanced, don't add excessive amounts of salt (sodium) to your food. Let the sodium and the potassium that is naturally found in foods be the main sources in your diet.

Magnesium is in bones and teeth and is needed for the orderly contraction of nerves and muscles. That is why its deficiency shows as muscle weakness and nervous instability.

Zinc helps the formation of hormones which regulate body growth and normal functions. Its deficiency leads to dwarfism, anemia, and slow healing of wounds.

You also need many other minerals, such as iodine for your thyroid and fluoride for your teeth. They are all in a balanced diet.

Our Nutritional Needs

Chapter 11

Nourishing the Baby
Till It Is Born

Following NutriScore is wise any time, but it is particularly so during pregnancy. You will notice that the rating level in most areas on the chart is higher for pregnant than for non-pregnant women. Remember to adjust your rating as soon as you know that you are pregnant.

Girls prepare physically for pregnancy from the day they themselves are conceived. The well-nourished fetus becomes a healthy, well-formed infant whose body, if properly fed, can produce in its turn healthy babies. Conversely, the children in populations where malnutrition prevails provide ample evidence in their poor bone structure, frequent physical and mental retardation, and susceptibility to disease that the nutritional sins of the mothers can indeed be visited upon the third and fourth generations. The sins of the fathers doubtless play their part, too; from the time the egg is fertilized until birth it is the mother upon whom the fetus depends for sustenance. If the mother herself is malnourished, things are off to a poor start, or even no start at all. Severe malnutrition is a known cause of miscarriage and stillbirth. Lifelong good nutrition is a woman's best preparation for pregnancy.

The first two weeks of pregnancy (the implantation stage) is a time when the mother's normal diet has great significance. Women often do not know that they are pregnant at this point and continue to eat according to their normal pattern. That's fine when the normal diet is adequate, because the increase in nutritional demands at first is minimal. But if the mother's diet is short on certain nutrients, she may be unable to supply even the fetus's modest requirements. If you are considering pregnancy, eat well, use alcohol and over-the-counter drugs sparingly, if at all, and follow the doctor's instructions for prescription drugs. Let him know immediately if you think you are pregnant, since some medical problems are handled with different medications during pregnancy; and you *know* you shouldn't smoke.

From two weeks to two months skeletal and organ development and differentiation are beginning in the fetus. Even though its needs are small, a poorly nourished woman without adequate stores of essential nutrients takes a chance on depriving her baby of the elements necessary to this development.

From eight weeks to term the growth and development of the fetus are rapid and the mother must increase her nutritional intake to fulfill the combined requirements of the baby's body and her own. We used to think that if there was a shortage of any nutrient, the fetus would be served first, and women resigned themselves to the loss of "a tooth for every baby," believing the baby would rob their bodies whenever supplies were short. This is not true; mother and baby can both be undernourished. To nurture her own body and that of the fetus during the last seven months of pregnancy a woman definitely needs to take in extra calories, protein, vitamin A, thiamin, niacin, riboflavin, pyridoxine, folate, vitamin B_{12}, vitamin C, vitamin D, and vitamin E, calcium, phosphorus, iron and magnesium. This is clearly shown in Appendices B, C, and D.

The pregnant teenager has an exceptional need to increase her nutrient intake at this time because in all likelihood she is still growing along with her unborn baby.

Nutritional management during pregnancy is ultimately the responsibility of a woman's doctor. He is the one with the scientific instruments to determine if the baby is growing sufficiently and whether pregnancy is proceeding normally. He has the knowledge to deal with the strange anemias and metabolic abnormalities that can arise during pregnancy. If a woman can't tolerate certain foods during pregnancy, she should be sure her doctor is aware of it, so that he can advise her on adequate replacements. If she has morning sickness to any extent, she should inform the doctor so he will realize there has been a nutritional loss. Doctors generally hand out printed lists of essential foods, prescribe vitamin and mineral supplements, and indicate a desirable weight gain.

If you are not happy with his recommendations, talk it over with him. A caring and knowledgeable doctor will often refer his patients to a dietitian or a nutritionist for individual counselling. We want to emphasize that your doctor knows *you* and that you should never deviate from his or her recommendations.

What to eat when you're pregnant? Milk is an important food for pregnant women. Four glasses daily will supply most of the needed calcium and vitamin D and almost half of the protein. Skim or partly skim milk is often recommended particularly if the pregnant woman has an overweight problem. It could eliminate about 300 calories from fat while keeping all the protein, calcium and B vitamins. Be sure that milk is enriched with vitamin D and, if skim milk, with vitamin A.

Women who are not in the habit of drinking milk may find the prospect of downing four glasses a day rather burdensome; however, they should be motivated to do it for their unborn baby. Skim milk, particularly, is so light that it is easier to drink frequently.

Some women may wish to flavor their milk with small amounts of coffee or chocolate syrup. We don't advise adding a lot of these flavorings. Chocolate syrup is rich in fat and sugar. Tomato soup may be mixed with skim milk for a hot or cold drink. Extra powdered skim milk may be added in cooking or in drinks, like milk shakes. If your palate is especially accustomed to whole milk, try this: mix 1 quart of 2% milk with 1 quart of reconstituted dry or liquid skim milk. Add ½ cup dry skim and mix well. (Or mix 1 L of 2% milk with 1 L of reconstituted dry or liquid skim milk. Add 125 mL dry skim and mix well.) Store in the refrigerator. It has more protein, less fat, 114 calories per glass, and a rich taste.

Meat, fish, or beans twice a day, eggs once a day, liver once a week should certainly be included in the pregnant mother's diet. All these foods are necessary, particularly for their content of protein and iron. Liver is very low in fat and for all the vitamins and iron it contains it is definitely worth including in the diet. In pregnancy, the mother's blood volume must increase and protein and iron are critical components of this increase.

Whole-grain or enriched cereals or bread should be eaten four times every day. These are well worth their cost for the calories, protein, iron, and B vitamins they contain.

Fruits and vegetables should be eaten at least four times a day to supplement adequate vitamins A and C and bulk in the diet. One of these should be citrus—orange or grapefruit or their juices. These are good sources of vitamin C. If you prefer, in the spring when they are plentiful, ten strawberries, or in the autumn, a half melon would do in place of citrus fruits. One serving should be a dark green or yellow vegetable, which is a particularly good source of vitamin A. Raw fruits and vegetables are encouraged. They can be eaten as snacks and desserts and help avoid excessive caloric intakes.

A vitamin/mineral supplement is often prescribed by doctors for pregnant women. This should be taken in exactly the prescribed dose.

Never take more than is prescribed. It is dangerous to think that if one is good, three or more will be that much better. It is also dangerous to consider these supplements as substitutes for a balanced diet. You get a lot more nutritional benefits from good food than you'll find in the most high-powered pill, so think of supplements as just that, something added to your diet.

Pregnancy is no time for dieting. The old wives' tale that a pregnant woman must eat for two was popular, but it led to overeating and overindulgence. A few decades ago, the medical profession went to the opposite extreme: restrict weight gain. Where is the truth? A careful review of the available research indicates that a maternal weight gain in the range of 20 to 25 pounds or 9 to 11 kg is needed for a better than average course of pregnancy. The patterns and rate of weight gain are particularly important. Sudden sharp weight gains and losses should be avoided at all cost. Gaining 2 pounds (or 1 kg) in the first three months or so, and one pound (or .5 kg) every 10 days for the rest of the pregnancy is considered "normal."

There is no scientific justification for the routine restriction of weight gain below 20 pounds (9 kg). Severe restriction of calories is potentially harmful to both mother and unborn infant. Even if the mother has a weight problem, severe restriction of calories is not desirable. It may mean that the unborn infant must use ketones, which are the debris from burning the mother's body fat, instead of the balanced nutrients from her diet.

Caloric restriction is also frequently accompanied by restrictions of nutrients essential for development, such as protein and iron. Researchers have linked severe caloric restrictions with low blood sugar, low levels of insulin, and high amino acid and ketone concentration in the blood of the mother. Weight reduction of obese women should be done either before or after pregnancy and dealt with under a physician's care.

Water is retained in larger amounts than usual during pregnancy because it is needed in the womb to guard the fetus against shocks, and in the blood to increase its volume. This increase in blood volume is needed to help move an unusual amount of waste and to carry oxygen and nourishment for the fetus. Many pregnant women have a small amount of swelling from water, a condition called edema. The doctor is the person to decide how much edema may be undesirable. The pregnant woman is not wise to limit her fluids or use a diuretic without medical advice.

Toxemia in pregnancy is manifested by edema (water retention) and is often accompanied by high blood pressure. It used to be thought that salt restriction, with or without a diuretic, was necessary for toxemia sufferers, but the recent trend has been towards making sure the patient takes in adequate protein, without particular concern about weight gain or retention of water. Toxemia is not a condition to fool around with, however, and if it's your doctor's considered opinion that you should restrict salt, restrict it. We know a mother who had toxemia before the birth of each of her three sons. She says she'd be willing to try once more for a girl, except that she can't face all those breakfasts of porridge and poached eggs without salt!

Morning sickness is thought to be caused by the newly formed fetus digging into the lining of the womb. It passes around the fourth month and until then the most common treatment is grin (or grimace) and bear it. Never take Gravol or other anti-nausea pills, unless they have been specifically prescribed by your doctor during that pregnancy. The period of morning sickness, unfortunately, is the time when there is most risk of medication crossing the placental barrier and damaging the developing fetus. There are lots of old tricks for combatting morning sickness, and you might experiment by drinking a cup of tea or glass of juice brought to your bed before rising, eating a piece of dry toast first thing, giving up coffee (coffee and bacon are notorious morning sickeners), and eating small meals more frequently rather than three large ones. Something's bound to help, if only the passage of time. Just be warned: "morning sickness" is a misnomer—it can strike anytime.

Indigestion and constipation often occur in the second half of pregnancy and reflect a reduction in acidity of the stomach and in the mobility of food through the gastro-intestinal tract. These are natural changes brought about by hormonal control that allows the food to remain longer in the gastro-intestinal tract in order to increase its utilization and absorption. To deal with these changes we recommend that the pregnant woman avoid fatty foods and favor a bland and bulky diet. It would also be helpful to eat smaller meals more frequently.

Nutritionally speaking, the emphasis during pregnancy should be on: (1) a weight gain of about 20 to 25 pounds (9 to 11 kg); (2) an adequate intake of protein; (3) a variety of foods in the diet including milk, cheese, eggs, meat, poultry, fish, beans, bread, cereals, fruits, and vegetables; and (4) a supplement of vitamins and minerals as prescribed by a physician.

REMEMBER

If you plan on getting pregnant some day, then it is essential that your diet rates well at all times. You need to start pregnancy in a well-nourished state and have full body reserves of protein, vitamins, and minerals.

Both mother and child will suffer the malnourishment of a mother with bad eating habits. Don't take chances, use foods from each group.

If you are not a milk drinker, this may be the time to get into the habit even if you have to flavor it or cook with it.

Notice as the pregnancy progresses that you will be more comfortable with smaller and more frequent meals. Still, make sure that you don't drift into eating junky snacks; keep score of your diet all the time.

If you have a weight problem, pregnancy is no time for dieting. Deal with your weight problem either before or after pregnancy, not during.

Go to a doctor who understands pregnant women and who is willing to discuss your problems with sympathy.

Chapter 12

Nourishing a Growing Body

The nursing mother requires most of the same nutrients she needed in the latter part of pregnancy, and even more calories. Intake should increase by about 1000 calories per day. This explains why many nursing mothers often find themselves hungry during the day. Those with a weight problem will find this a particularly good time to reduce. They can return to normal physical activity and without having to apply rigid control over their diet can shed unwanted pounds.

The need for iron, folate, and vitamin B_{12} in the nursing mother is at about the same level as for the non-pregnant female. The need for other vitamins and minerals and protein for lactation is about the same as for pregnancy.

A daily eating plan should include six glasses of milk (preferably skim), two servings of meat, fish or beans, one egg, four servings of whole-grain or enriched cereals or bread, and four servings of fruits and vegetables (one from those listed in each of areas C, D, E, and F of the rating chart in Chapter 2). In addition, physicians often prescribe a vitamin and mineral supplement for the nursing mother and some-times for the infant. In either case, the dose recommended by the physician should never be exceeded.

This diet plan is similar to that suggested for pregnancy except it has two extra glasses of milk. The milk formula suggested for pregnancy may be used here. Additional foods are needed to meet the caloric needs but these could vary depending on the desirability of weight gain or loss of the mother.

There has been a definite trend away from breast feeding and towards prepared baby formulas throughout the world in the past few decades. This is unfortunate for developing countries that have poor sanitation, illiteracy (and therefore, little information about nutrition), poverty, unequal distribution of food, and inadequate weaning diets. The decline of breast feeding in such countries applies across all socio-economic classes.

In industrialized countries, the trend towards baby formula occurs mainly in lower-income groups. The current trend among the upper-income and well-educated groups of the wealthier countries is increasingly towards breast feeding.

The case for the superiority of breast milk over other forms of feeding is based on the nutrient components of human milk, its convenience, its economy, its psychological benefits, and its anti-infective properties. All of the arguments in favor of nursing can be countered except this last. Breast milk, particularly in the first month or so, contains desirable friendly bacteria that check the growth of dangerous bacteria in the baby's intestine, as well as valuable anti-bodies that fight disease-causing germs. This is particularly valuable in protecting the baby in the early weeks; in time the bottle-fed baby gets his own immune system working. The North American mother who is unable to nurse her baby should pay special attention to the cleanliness and sanitation of the baby's environment. In developing countries where sanitary conditions are poor the practice of breast feeding has been found to greatly reduce the incidence of diarrhea.

Cow's milk can, when necessary, simulate human milk. To achieve this: (1) the protein is treated to produce a softer, more flocculent curd that is digested more easily by the infant; (2) the milk is diluted to reduce the calcium level to that of human milk. (3) dialysis may be used to reduce the sodium content to equal that of human milk; (4) butterfat may be removed in part and vegetable oil or oils added to increase the amount of polyunsaturated fatty acid, especially linoleic acid. Fat in this form best imitates the fat content of human milk and it is best tolerated by the infant.

Most of the commercial formulas seem adequate, although we wouldn't choose one listing coconut or palm oil among the ingredients. They are saturated fats that provide little or no linoleic acid. We would also avoid ready-to-feed preparations with emulsifiers and stabilizers added to them. We prefer reconstituting the powder form. Remember to use water that has been boiled for 20 minutes, then cooled.

Many mothers may be interested in nursing their babies for several weeks or a few months. This is reasonable. The baby may be given a bottle of formula once a day or two or three times a week in addition to breast feeding.

Alternatively, breast feeding may continue for the better part of a year if the mother and baby find it satisfying and satisfactory. In many developing countries, breast feeding may go on for two or more years.

The psychological and emotional advantages of breast feeding to both mother and child are important factors. A great deal of work with animals has indicated that early feeding experience does affect behavior. In the long term, however, behavior is affected by many factors and the precise role of the feeding method cannot be pinpointed clearly in human infants. It is up to the mother to assess her whole situation and decide how nursing the baby will affect the maternal and familial relationship.

As the baby grows his vitamins, minerals, and protein will come from a variety of foods to supplement the breast or bottled milk. Depending upon the baby and the doctor, sometime in the first half of the first year—probably about the fourth month—such supplementary foods as cereals, egg yolk, stewed strained fruits and vegetables, and strained meats appear on the infant's menu. Iron, vitamin C, and vitamin D are the nutrients most needed in supplementation. The doctor will probably prescribe vitamin D in chemical form, iron in the form of strained meats (in particular, liver), and orange juice for vitamin C.

As new foods are introduced the baby may react unfavorably with indigestion, diarrhea, constipation, or allergic responses such as exzema. For this reason new foods should be offered one at a time and in small amounts. In the event that a baby does not tolerate a food well, consult your doctor.

Usually, pediatricians suggest solid foods by the second month; some earlier and some later. We feel this is too early to start most babies on solid food, especially breast-fed babies. It tends to encourage overeating, which may lead to fat babies and fat adults with many complications later on in life. Unless the baby has a special eating problem, solid foods could be safely delayed till the fourth month. Your doctor should be able to give you the best advice. The first food suggested is cereal. This is because milk, breast or bottle, is low in iron, and by then the iron reserves the baby is born with soon diminish. Try one cereal at a time to detect any allergies. Start with a rice cereal; it is rare that babies are allergic to rice. Try barley next, then oatmeal, and after that you may try mixed cereals. In choosing a baby cereal, always pick one that has little or no sugar, salt, or hydrogenated fat.

By the third or fourth month, you should be able also to give the baby strained vegetables, such as squash, beans, broccoli, and carrots; again one at a time to detect allergies, if they occur. A month later, start introducing strained fruits such as bananas, peaches, applesauce, and apricots, also one at a time. By introducing vegetables first, you get the baby accustomed to their taste; an excellent eating habit to form that will pay dividends all through life. Often, if you introduce fruits first, the baby will become so accustomed to sweetness that he may refuse vegetables.

Vegetables and fruits are rich sources of vitamin A and C and other vitamins. In fact, your doctor will advise you to introduce strained orange juice for its vitamin C quite early, often by the end of the second month or the start of the third month.

By month five or six, mashed and strained egg yolk is introduced as an additional source of iron, protein, and a variety of vitamins and minerals. Egg white is not given to babies at this time since many develop an allergy to it at this early age. Most pediatricians wouldn't recommend giving whole eggs until the baby is about nine months old.

By the sixth or seventh month, the baby will be ready for strained meat. The variety in the baby's diet and the balance of nutrients in all these foods will certainly insure his or her health and nourishment. Think of it—the baby will be having milk, cereals, vegetables, fruits, egg, and meat.

Gradually, and within a few months, babies become accustomed to coarser foods. The diet changes from puréed to chopped food.

By seven months of age, the baby usually is able to pick up foods in his hands, and suck and munch on them, as well as spread them over his face, hair, clothes, and the furniture. The first tooth is usually breaking through at this time. Crusts of bread or teething biscuits are particularly satisfying to suck and chew on.

Lumpier foods may be allowed so that they can be picked up by the fingers as the baby feeds himself or herself more and more. Meats, however, should still be ground and minced fine, as they are usually hard for very small children to chew.

Eating at the family table makes this changeover relatively easy for the baby. It may, however, be nerve-racking for the parents. But, from there on, things improve. More teeth spring out. Muscle co-ordination improves, and gradually the baby learns to handle eating utensils. The dietary scope expands from dependency on milk alone to a list that contains literally hundreds of items. Within a very short span of time, we have gone through weaning, baby foods, junior foods to adult food, and before long, he or she is a baby no more.

Commercially prepared baby and junior foods are hygienic. The sanitary standards are usually strict and well controlled. Commercially prepared products also help the mother save time. Their labels list nutrients to help compare nutritional values. They also list ingredients—apricots, cornstarch, salt—which is helpful in preventing allergic reactions.

There was a time when baby foods were sweetened, salted, and sometimes flavored. They were made to appeal to the mother's taste buds, not the baby's. A baby has no inborn yearning for added salt or sweetness or for such exotic flavors as chocolate. He is perfectly happy to take his food *au naturel* until he is taught to do otherwise. It is the mother to whom plain, unsalted, uncreamed, unsweetened spinach tastes peculiar, and the manufacturers operated on the basis that she buys most readily the products seasoned for the adult palate.

It is a welcome development that so many commercially prepared baby foods now declare on the label 'no salt added' and 'no sugar added'. These should be our choice, not the ones that are salted and sugared. A high salt intake can be hard on the infant's kidneys, throw the body into a negative water balance and aggravate a familial predisposition towards hypertension. Excessive sugaring of foods will program our children to expect sweetness in many foods and lead to high sugar consumption throughout life. This has undesirable effects on teeth and gums, encourages fat deposits in the body, and aggravates a familial predisposition towards diabetes.

There are times when commercial baby foods are your best bet. Commercially prepared strained beef liver, heart, lamb, or poultry with nothing added are wholesome and quick. Simple strained vegetables such as peas, beans, and carrots without sugar and starch (if possible) are useful when you're rushed. Simple fruits like applesauce and peaches can be recommended although they have sugar added. Avoid those with tapioca and starch added because you will be paying fruit prices for starch. Fortified infant cereals without sugar or fruits offer more than any cereal you can prepare at home. And for those days when you're extra busy, or traveling or, heaven forbid, sick, the comfort of knowing that there's a meal for baby ready at the twist of a screw-cap is indescribable.

On the other hand, for some foods, home-cooking is best. All you need are standard kitchen utensils, including an inexpensive fine mesh strainer. A blender, food processor, and pressure cooker are handy but not essential. Do pay particular attention to cleanliness. All utensils must be sterilized in boiling water before each use. If you stew your own fruit and freeze it in small ice cube containers you know what's in it. Apples, peaches, pears, apricots, and prunes are the best fruits to stew for babies. Bananas don't need cooking; they can be scraped or well-mashed and served raw.

Vegetables, likewise, may be prepared at home and frozen in individual servings. These include peas, tomatoes, squash, carrots, beets, string beans, spinach, and sweet potatoes. Corn is discouraged because of its tough husks. Even strongly flavored vegetables such as cabbage, cauliflower, turnips, and broccoli may be tried after boiling with two water changes. Don't worry about the losses of vitamins and minerals in the boiling water; you can use the water for soup stock and there will be enough left to make it worthwhile. It will help the baby develop good eating habits to be introduced to these flavors at an early age.

Eggs may be hard-cooked. Babies under eight or nine months of age should be given only the yolk since they may develop allergies to the egg white. In this case, separate the yolk.

Foods to avoid include nuts, raw peas, berries, and other small but firm foods that can be swallowed the wrong way, causing the baby to choke. Chocolate and cocoa are not necessary and are likely to cause allergies. Candy is of no particular nutritional value, causes tooth decay, and leads to poor eating habits. Under no circumstances should candy be given as a bribe or a reward for good behavior or for eating other foods. You couldn't hurt your child's eating habits more than when you dangle candy before him or her. Sweet cookies, cakes, and pastries should not be offered frequently. They are detrimental to the teeth and gums and are not balanced foods.

The eating habits of our children and teenagers are below par. Studies in both the United States and Canada have pointed to a number of deficiencies in the diets of children and adolescents. In a study by the Child Research Council in the United States, the diets of only half the boys examined between one and 10 years of age contained the recommended dietary allowances. A study of the diets of over 3000 pre-school children showed them low in fruits and vegetables and high in candy, soft drinks, pastries, and fried snacks. According to Nutrition Canada, a third or more of children and adolescents in Canada had diets low in iron, about a quarter of them were low in calcium, and one out of six were low in vitamin C.

Children and adolescents need more of each nutrient in relation to their body size than adults do. Their growing bodies need building blocks. Also, they are more active and the body needs fuel.

Physical growth proceeds according to a specific pattern. We see the fastest growth, both in weight and in height, in the first year of life and in the early teens. On the whole, girls develop earlier than boys. But boys and girls vary individually. Some grow fast in the early teens, others do not achieve their maximum growth until they are 15 to 17 years. At times they eat an enormous amount of food and put on weight in an alarming fashion. Then, they shoot upward and go back to their slim, attractive, healthy-looking selves.

Physical activity is an important factor in the nourishment of children and teenagers. Active kids eat more to compensate the body for energy spent. The more food they eat, the more nutrients they get and the less likely they are to become deficient (assuming poor eating habits don't lead them to rely heavily on junk foods). Almost always, the active child is more likely to be well-nourished than the sedentary, quiet child.

The impact of poor eating habits among children and adolescents shows in a variety of ways. In its severest forms, malnutrition may affect growth and learning ability. This is an extreme case. More commonly, one may observe listlessness and inability to concentrate in school among children who eat little or no breakfast. Susceptibility to infections and continual fatigue are likely to be observed, particularly among adolescent girls on bizarre reducing diets. Children and adolescents on poor diets do not enjoy the best chance for physical and mental development, and poor diets may well predispose them to health problems in their adult years.

How can we ensure good eating habits in young people? Eating habits, like any other habits are formed early in life. Since eating is a frequent and regular activity, these habits are enforced and become set at a very early age. So, examine the eating practices in your family. None of us is perfect, and if nutrition has been somewhat slighted at your house, take the attitude "better late than never" and start today. After all, you're going to be eating for the rest of your life, so you may as well do it right.

A few concrete suggestions:

Parents should not skip meals. The critical meal in this regard is breakfast. While adults may get away without it for a while, eventually their liveliness, stamina, and productivity are affected; children should never get the idea that they can go without breakfast.

Serve meals at regular hours set for the convenience of the parents and the feeding schedule of the children. Everyone should be mildly hungry, not starved, and not overtired. This may mean a sizable snack for the children to carry them to mealtime or parents arriving home at a reasonable time before meals so that they can relax before eating. If they are both working and arrive home too tired to cope, it might be a good idea to take turns resting for 10 minutes before mealtime.

Feed young children first. This does not mean the children should be allowed to rush through the meal. Parents can slow down their children's eating by engaging them in conversation (or motions and play if the children are too young to talk).

Don't worry about day-to-day variations in children's appetites. Some days they will eat well, others they will not. The children should never be coaxed into cleaning their plates. It is best not to comment on a young child's eating habits, either positively or negatively. Eating need not be rewarded, nor should eating little be punished. The important thing is to serve firmly and repeatedly a variety of nutritious foods and not to give in to demands for foods of little nutritional value. We can be permissive with our children on many issues in order to allow them to develop mentally, socially, and intellectually. When it comes to nutrition, there is no place for permissiveness.

"If vegetables were candies, my kids would eat them." We hear complaints like this all the time from parents who are resigned to the fact that their children were born with a dislike of vegetables that is unshakable. This is untrue.

What is required is a firm, positive parental attitude. Remember that vitamins, minerals, other nutrients, and roughage come from vegetables. Youngsters are copycats, of course. If Dad puts up a fuss whenever squash is brought to the table, the children will do the same. Either Dad must change or other vegetables (see areas E and F of the rating chart in Chapter 2) should be substituted.

While the children are young offer raw vegetables with meals and between meals to start them on healthful eating habits. A hunk of cucumber on a hot day or a stalk of celery are good and satisfying snacks for a young child and don't destroy his appetite.

Add extra vegetables to a stew or a soup if you feel that dinner with separate vegetables becomes a battlefield too often. Canned, prepared soups are beloved by most children and they can be made even more nourishing by the addition of extra vegetables. In fact, some of these quick convenience products like canned soups, spaghetti, and macaroni make fine lunches for youngsters, particularly if you use them as vehicles for extra vegetables.

Salads are in a class by themselves and you should feature them each day. We learned, very early, that busy professionals who are parents are often too tired in the evening to prepare a full meal plus salad for the family. Here is where the kids can help. Making a salad themselves is the best method we know to interest kids from 5 to 95 in eating greens at every meal.

Learning to cook will insure that kids learn to eat properly. Salad making is a good place to start. Work with them to master weekend morning muffins, then on to simple casseroles and hamburgers.

By 10 years, some of the youngsters we know can help prepare a meal, and by 12 they are well on their way to sharing equally in the work of the kitchen.

It is impossible to overstate the case for parental control in the eating habits of their children. Remain friendly but firm. Love your kids as you deny them pops and fries. Be consistent. Don't allow junk foods, whatever the occasion.

Try not to become hung up on the children's use of utensils and their general table manners. It is more sensible to set the example rather than turn mealtime conversation into a session of "do this" and "don't do that."

As children enter the teenage years, remember that social influences affect their thinking and behavior. Nutrition habits should not be a matter of controversy and debate, otherwise they will become a subject of parental defiance. Parents may continue to influence their children's eating habits in subtle ways by firmly excluding foods and beverages of low nutritional value from their shopping list, and by adopting good eating habits for themselves (regular meal hours, not skipping breakfast, large variety of foods, milk with some meals, good snacking habits and eating modest amounts). When your teenager points out to you that you don't drink enough milk with your meals, you should take the hint and take pride that he or she knows about good nutrition.

Parents should encourage sports, fitness and exercise for themselves and their children. Encourage them to take up as many sports as their school program allows. Invest in sports clothes and equipment. Have the whole family participate in the local Y programs. Take time for sports and/or recreation activity with your teenagers and their friends (for as long as they accept you among them!).

Not only is physical activity valuable to health but it allows the body better physiological control on appetite. Studies showed that active people regulate their caloric intake to match their energy expenditure more accurately than do sedentary people. Thus, active people are not as likely to become obese. This increased activity should be encouraged, particularly among teenage girls who tend to be preoccupied with weight control, go on crash or fad diets and often subject themselves to a definite health hazard.

In the teenage years, the more active the person, the more he or she eats, the better the chances are that the diet will supply the protein, vitamins and minerals needed. Exercise increases the need for calories but not for protein, vitamins, and minerals. Active adolescents are healthier and are likely to be better nourished than inactive ones. Don't forget also that active teenagers are likely to have a better self-image. Their bodies are well-developed. They are slim, have good musculature, and their bones are straight. These are important attributes to a teenager.

Parents can do a lot to cultivate good eating habits in their children. But, let's face it, our children spend most of their waking hours at school. Many of our children eat at least one meal and possibly two snacks a day at school. As parents, it is our business to examine the schools' food service facilities and practices.

Neither parents nor teachers should tolerate junk foods in schools. Vending machines dispensing pop, candies, and chips should be converted to serve milk, fruit juices, muffins, buns, biscuits, apples, and oranges. Rich desserts, fried foods, soft drinks, and candies should not be allowed in school cafeterias and snack bars. School boards in Bloomington, Indiana; Washington, D.C.; Dallas, Texas; and Montreal, Quebec, have already acted to outlaw sugar-loaded foods or require vendors to include some nutritious foods in machines placed in the schools. No doubt many other school boards will follow suit.

Nutrition should be taught in all schools. It is a subject matter that can have the most profound impact on the future of our children. The food service practices in the school should enforce the subject taught in the classroom. Students should be allowed to apply what they learn about nutrition to the operation of the school's cafeteria and vending machines.

Every member of the family deserves a say in menu-planning. We can't tell you exactly what to eat because a proper diet varies according to a person's needs and likes and dislikes. Get each member of your family to rate his or her diet on the rating chart in Chapter 2. Then try to improve everyone's score with regard to his or her preferences in the foods in each area of the chart. It shouldn't be too hard to make every meal "good eating" in both the nutritional and the aesthetic sense.

REMEMBER

If you are able, breast feed your baby even for the first few weeks. It is better than not at all. Nothing beats mother's milk in its nutritional value, its convenience, its economy, its psychological benefits, and its anti-infective quality.

If you cannot breast feed your baby for some physiological or psychological reason, consult your doctor on choosing a formula where the protein has been treated to a soft, flocculent curd, the salts have been dialyzed and diluted to the levels of human milk, the source of fat is polyunsaturated, and the necessary vitamins and minerals have been added to the levels in human milk.

If you are breast feeding your baby, and often even if you are bottle feeding, chances are that you will not need to introduce solid foods until the fourth month. Discuss it with your doctor, but resist any attempts to put the baby on solid foods too early.

Introduce foods one at a time to allow any possible allergies to develop and be traced to specific food. Then you will know what to avoid in the future.

Prepare your own baby food without adding salt, sugar, or starches. Prepare it carefully and preserve it properly.

When you buy commercial baby foods, choose the ones that don't list such ingredients as salt, sugar, starch, and non-food sounding names. Ignore desserts and complete dinners. Your baby is better off without them.

As your baby becomes a child and a teenager, work on his or her eating habits. Emphasize wholesome foods and discourage ones with little value. Even if you know that soda pop is available at the corner store and candies are bought at the variety shop, don't put them on your shopping list or allow them in your house. Always explain your position. There is no room for permissiveness when it comes to nutrition. Stick to your principles, follow them yourself, and never give in to children's pressure. Some day they will appreciate you for it.

Chapter 13
Nutrition Without Growth

The nutritional needs of adults differ from those of children and adolescents. As adults become less active physically, their caloric needs decline. Their blood volume does not increase. Therefore, the iron needs for men drop slightly due to good conservation of iron stored in the body. Iron needs for women stay high to compensate for menstrual blood losses. Since the body skeleton ceases growing in adult years, the calcium, phosphorus, vitamin D, and fluoride needs drop slightly from the levels in childhood and adolescence. The needs for protein, vitamins, and minerals involved in life processes do not change.

The main concern for adults is to be active so that caloric needs do not drop to a point that makes it difficult to eat well. While keeping rich desserts and fried foods to a minimum, grown-ups may well shift, if they haven't already, from whole or partly skimmed (2%) to totally skimmed milk.

A daily eating plan should include two glasses of skim milk, two servings of meat, fish, or beans, one egg or an ounce of cheese (on alternate days), four servings of fruits and vegetables (one from those listed in each of areas, C, D, E and F of the NutriScore chart) and two servings of whole-grain or enriched bread or cereals (area G of the chart).

The great misconception among adults is that for them nutrition is no longer important since they are not growing anymore. This is not so. They need to cut down on their calories as they cut down on their physical activity, but maintain high intakes of protein, vitamins, and minerals.

A change in the body means a change in the diet. If you've lost teeth through an accident or poor oral health, you may have difficulty eating tough foods. Also, problems with digestion and absorption may mean that certain foods will disagree with you. Don't just drop such foods—find substitutes of similar nutritional value. Look in the NutriScore chart for a replacement. That is, unless the disallowed foods are rich desserts, fatty meats, fried snack foods, or soft drinks—those you may relinquish with never a moment's thought.

Women are more poorly nourished than men. On the face of it that fact, which has emerged from many nutrition surveys, is surprising. After all, women probably have more nutrition information than men, since they are the ones who do most of the cooking and feed most of the children in the country. There are several reasons to explain why they come out so poorly.

First, women need more of some nutrients, like iron. Second, women's body nutritional stores should be higher in the event of pregnancy. Their nutrition status is crucial. Third, women tend to subject themselves to severe dieting more often than men. They are generally not as active as men and they are given to crash diets, skipping meals or complete fasting in order to lose weight in a hurry.

Living alone can be a traumatic social and nutritional experience whether you are young or old, a college student in a rooming house or a businessman on the road. Single, separated, and widowed people all lead this living-alone pattern of having to shop, prepare, and eat food for one. Often, it is so discouraging that meals become haphazard.

A serious problem confronting these lone people is in shopping for food. Mostly all items are packaged for families. Without careful planning, you may end up with a lot of wasted leftovers, wilted vegetables and rotten fruits. Stock up on frozen vegetables so that you can take what you need and keep the rest in the freezer. Buy the individually wrapped frozen fish fillets and separate them one at a time without thawing the whole package. Divide your loaf of bread, use what you will eat for two days at a time and freeze the rest. Shop at fruit and vegetable markets where you can pick the amounts you need and not get stuck with a prepackaged supply for a family of five or six. Whatever you do, fight any tendencies to boredom and tired indifference towards food.

Unwise dieting constitutes a severe insult to the body, which often bears the marks. Not long ago, we met a young woman in her early twenties who was a bit on the heavy side but not grossly obese. Her complexion lacked the normal pinkish tone of the human flesh. Her breakfast used to consist of a two-ounce bag (60 g) of hard candy. It contained 220 calories, zero of protein or any of the vitamins or minerals. She was on a diet that gave her for breakfast the one thing she needed to cut down on, calories, and nothing else. For the same number of calories, she could have had a small glass of orange juice, a piece of toast, even a little butter and jam, and a glass of skim milk. This would have supplied a quarter of her daily needs of protein, more than half her calcium needs, a third of her needs of thiamin and riboflavin and all her needs for vitamin C for the day. It is senseless dieting that leads to malnutrition, ill health, and what may bother the dieter most of all, a poor appearance.

Obesity appears to be the most common nutritional problem among adults in North America. Estimates suggest that one in two in Canada to one in three in the U.S. are suffering from some degree of overweight. The proportion of obese adults increases with age in both men and women. This suggests that physical activity is an important factor. As a person grows older, his or her activity declines and unless the caloric intake drops proportionately, obesity will follow. It is a result of taking in more calories than are put out. In other words, it stems from eating too much or exercising too little. Most often it is a combination of both.

Obesity develops over a period of time and therefore does not shock the individual into doing something about it until it is advanced. If it were to come on rather suddenly, like other diseases, with an overnight gain of 20 pounds (90 kg), the impact would be dramatic and the individual would be shocked into finding out what he or she had done wrong and correcting the situation.

Obese people differ from non-obese people in two basic ways. First, the obese person is likely to eat in response to seeing, smelling, or thinking of food. The non-obese person eats because his body needs the fuel for work. Second, the obese person eats until the food supply is gone, while the non-obese person eats until his hunger is satisfied.

The ability of the body to regulate its appetite to match caloric intake with output is better controlled in people who are physically active. Studies with animals and humans show that those who are active spend more calories and eat to match the calories spent. They, therefore, do not accumulate abnormal amounts of fat. On the other hand, sedentary people do not spend many calories yet they tend to eat slightly more than they spend and accumulate fat deposits in their bodies.

It doesn't take much to become obese over a period of time. If, for example, you got into the habit of having an extra sliver of pie every day, that will amount to 200 extra calories a day which will put on 20 pounds (90 kg) per year. This, over a three-year period, would mean 60 pounds or 270 kg over what you started with.

What other foods would give you 200 calories? A generous shot of hard liquor, a bottle of beer, a half-inch slice of chocolate cake, two small doughnuts, or 15 potato chips.

Statistically, a grossly overweight person is at a high risk of death from cardiovascular and renal diseases, diabetes, liver and gall bladder diseases. An obese person has been giving his body more fuel than it needs. The body can't dump these calories, so it stores them as fat. Fat tissues expand, enzymes involved in making fat become active. Since making fat is tied to making other substances, there is increased metabolic capacity in the body. As a result, obesity leads to other strains on the body.

Obesity is an important contributing cause of heart attack and coronary heart disease, because the obese person, as a result of eating more than normal, has more cholesterol and other fatty substances to deposit along the walls of the blood vessels. When this occurs the blood vessels harden, thus losing their ability to expand and contract flexibly with heartbeats. They thicken internally, sometimes to the extent that they block the free circulation of the blood. The result of these changes can be a heart attack or coronary heart disease.

High blood cholesterol appears to be directly linked to high consumption of saturated fat and cholesterol. This is an area of much debate among nutrition scientists, but through all the controversies there are clear indications that your blood cholesterol rises when you eat more saturated fat, less polyunsaturated fat and/or more cholesterol. By the same token, the way to lower blood cholesterol is to cut down on fat consumption, to eat less saturated and more poly-unsaturated fats, and to lower your consumption of cholesterol-rich foods.

All of the evidence from long-term studies on populations shows that high blood cholesterol, especially those of the low density lipoproteins (LDL) in the blood, are related to the incidence of coronary heart disease. The relationship is continuous, so there is hardly a point above or below which the risk of a heart attack suddenly increases or decreases. The evidence is so compelling that the development of sensible dietary habits becomes imperative.

We do not advocate the complete elimination of certain foods from the diet. It is a matter of adjustment of quantities consumed. For example, in the North American diet, well over 40 per cent of the calories come from fat. When we correlate the level of fat calories in various countries with deaths from coronary heart disease we find that the incidence increases sharply with the increase of dietary fat above 30 per cent of the diet calories. So, we need to lower the fat in our diet from well over 40 per cent to 30 per cent or less. We need to cut our fat intake by about a quarter of its present amount. Our efforts should be directed to avoiding foods in area H of the NutriScore chart, cutting down on rich desserts, trimming the fat from steaks, drinking skim milk instead of whole milk, substituting low fat dressings for high fat ones, using less butter on bread and less mayonnaise in our sandwiches and salads.

There is strong scientific evidence in favor of increasing the proportion of polyunsaturated fat over that of saturated fat in the diet. This doesn't mean to completely eliminate saturated fat. In general, animal fat is higher in saturated fat than in polyunsaturated fat, except in the case of oily fish like herring and sardines. On the other hand, vegetable oils are higher in polyunsaturated than in saturated fats, with the exception of coconut oil, which is a saturated fat. This is important to remember since coconut oil is added to many foods. When it is, you will find it on the list of ingredients on the label. We recommend that, as much as possible, you use oils more than shortening, lard or butter for cooking. Among commercially available vegetable oils, safflower, and corn oils have higher polyunsaturated to saturated fat ratios than most. In place of butter or margarine, we recommend you prepare your own blended butter from butter and oil according to the formula we gave in Chapter 4 of this book.

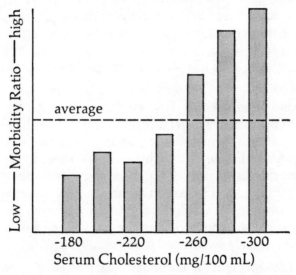

The risk of coronary heart disease in men 30 to 49 years old, in a 14-year study conducted in Framingham, Massachussets.

North Americans should eat fewer cholesterol-containing foods. At the moment their diet is estimated to include half a gram or more of cholesterol. It would be desirable to reduce this amount by about half. This is difficult because some foods that are high in cholesterol are also high in nutritional quality and should not be eliminated completely from the diet except on a doctor's advice. Examples are eggs and liver. In spite of their cholesterol content, we recommend that pregnant women and nursing mothers should include one egg a day and three ounces (85 g) of liver a week in their diet. Older children, adolescents and adults may do with only three eggs and two ounces (60 g) of liver per week. This is providing that the person is not under other specific instructions from a physician. Milk is not overly rich in cholesterol by comparison with eggs but even that little bit may be cut down or eliminated by drinking partly skim or skim milk. Some foods high in cholesterol that need not form a habitual part of the diet are brain, caviar, and shellfish such as oysters, lobster, shrimp, and crab. They may be eaten on occasion, but don't make them a habit.

A reduction in our consumption of sugar can only be beneficial. Sugar provides empty calories. We can get the same energy plus numerous useful nutrients from many other foods. Moreover, some people are genetically predisposed to increase their blood cholesterol from high consumption of table sugar. In those individuals, part of the sugar molecule appears to favor increased formation of fat and cholesterol in the body. Also, for those who are diabetic or predisposed to diabetes, high consumption of sugar and other carbohydrates presents a specific hazard. These individuals should be under medical care. Our recommendation for everyone else is moderate use of sugar. Attempt to use it less and less, particularly in situations where you tend to "dish" it out, as in coffee or tea, on breakfast cereals and on desserts.

High blood pressure, or hypertension is a strong risk in the development of coronary heart disease. Many studies have shown this.

For a long time scientists have observed a consistent relationship between high salt intake and high blood pressure. Recent studies on monkeys indicated that not only high salt but the combination of high salt and sugar in the diet increases the magnitude of hypertension and the risk of coronary heart disease. Should this turn out to apply to humans as well, our concern over the dangers of a diet with highly salted and excessively sweetened foods would be justified.

Dietary management of coronary heart disease is only part of a complex prevention or treatment system. During the adult years much effort should be directed to controlling high blood pressure and emotional and mental stresses, cutting out or down on smoking, and increasing physical fitness.

Our Western civilization has spawned a lifestyle that combines all these evils. The more we advance in our careers the less physical work we are likely to do and the more office-bound we become. Mental stress becomes a way of life as we work late hours, skip or delay meals, and drive everyone in the office ruthlessly to get things done. We are also expected to be on the road most of the time. We have to be mobile if we are to get things done. This means over-eating on expense accounts, breaking a secure and often needed routine of life and getting little or no chance for relaxation or recreation.

If for one reason or another, we cannot completely change business demands on our time, we could slightly alter them for the better. Small meals throughout the day would be one suggestion; and if the 5 o'clock meeting threatens to run until 10 at night, we should take time for a glass of milk and a sandwich, a piece of cheese and fruit or another small but nourishing snack. We know a successful businessman who made a habit, whenever a meeting ran long and tense, to excuse himself and step out for a breath of fresh air or to run up and down the staircase for three or four stories to overcome, as he put it, "the tardiness of the mind."

Executives are not alone in choosing food patterns that are potential killers. It truly disturbs us to see whole families just asking for trouble with their orders for milk shakes, chocolate sundaes, and chips all round. "All round" will soon describe the people who eat like that. People manage their money with an eye to tomorrow, yet they'll squander their physical resources. And yet we know that tomorrow's good health is the one thing tomorrow's money can't buy. We have to pay into that account a little bit every day of our lives.

REMEMBER

As adults, we bear the marks of our nutritional backgrounds. But most problems can be dealt with by adequate nutrition arrangement.

The one thing you must watch for as an adult is staying active. Keep your calories burning. Don't lay on fat and deposit cholesterol in your arteries.

If you haven't cut down on fat, especially animal fat and coconut or palm oil (they are saturated), it is never too late to start. Trim the fat off your meat. Boil, poach or bake food rather than fry it. Limit eggs to three or four a week and liver to once a week, but don't drop them completely.

Remember the dietary guidelines to eat a variety of foods; to maintain ideal weight; to avoid too much fat, saturated fat, and cholesterol; to eat foods with adequate starch and fiber; to avoid too much sugar; to avoid too much sodium; and, if you drink alcohol, to do so in moderation.

Chapter 14

Growing Old, Healthy and Happy

More people are living now well past retirement than in any other time in history. Almost 8 per cent of the population in Canada and the U.S. are over 65 years of age. The figure fifty years ago was only 5 per cent. Our longevity today is a direct result of the many advances in medicine, particularly in the discovery of micro-organisms and the origin of infectious diseases. The development of sulpha drugs and antibiotics and their mass production have led to the eradication of many infectious diseases. Now we are living long enough to become victims of faulty diets.

Our nutritional needs do not change drastically upon retirement. We become less active and our basic metabolic rate decreases and, as a result, we require fewer calories. Therefore we have to eat less.

Women's iron needs decrease after the menopause because the menstrual blood loss (blood contains iron) is eliminated and iron stores need not be as high as is required for pregnancy.

Other than these two changes there is virtually no difference in the requirement for protein and most of the vitamins and minerals in the latter years than in the earlier years of adulthood.

So, it is just as important as ever for older people to keep on testing their diets and balancing them out on the NutriScore chart. The rating levels in each area will help you get a varied nutritious diet. The chart also offers alternative foods in each area in case you have to drop some of your favorite foods because of chewing or digestive difficulties.

A daily eating plan for an older person should include a glass or two of milk, a serving or two of meat, fish, chicken, or beans, an egg or an ounce of cheese (on alternative days), four servings of fruits and vegetables (one from those listed in each of areas C, D, E, and F of the rating chart in Chapter 2), and two servings of whole-grain or enriched bread or cereals.

Needless to say, the choice of foods and the way they should be prepared should take into account the difficulty older people often have chewing and digesting certain foods. Any dish you prepare should be properly cooked and if necessary strained. Foods that don't agree with you should be replaced with ones of equal nutritional value. Locate the food that you can no longer tolerate in one of the rating chart areas and select one of more substitutes in the same area.

Social and psychological problems in the golden years can interfere with good nutrition. In our society there is a strong link between social level and job status. A person who has struggled through a successful career and reached the top or close to it will attach a great deal of emotion to his achievement. Retirement can represent a loss in status and an emotional anti-climax. To many, the beginning of a new search for identity can be traumatic.

These latter years also represent the time when the children have left home. For women who devoted all their energies to motherhood this loss of the family circle creates a vacuum in their lives that leaves them victims of depression and feelings of inadequacy. Often they sink into a lethargy that disdains both exercise and food.

The loss of one's spouse also creates a tremendous vacuum. The golden years abruptly lose their shine. The surviving partner often moves from the family home to smaller and more manageable quarters, and the loss of friends and familiar surroundings can be upsetting enough to result in a disinterest in his or her own health.

For many, retirement also means a serious financial strain on a fixed income. If one considers the longevity statistics of North Americans, it becomes evident that the chances are greater for the husband to die before his wife. Think of the enormous social, psychological, and financial strain many women face in the latter years of life.

The impact of these strains on nutrition and health is far-reaching. Mental depression and feelings of boredom, loss and emptiness, are likely to lead to loss of appetite. A woman who used to cook for a large appreciative family is not likely to plan meals as well or as enthusiastically for just herself.

Older people living alone have problems in shopping for food. The packaging of many foods is oriented towards a family unit (very few items are packaged for individual servings). Furthermore, they have difficulty carrying large bags and, therefore, may have to do their shopping in frequent trips, rather than once a week as they used to. Find a fruit store that will deliver and make up a weekly order of staples. (You can't blame them for not wanting to bring you four oranges and a pint of milk, but if you order your week's potatoes, toilet paper, lettuce, and so on, it will add up to enough to make a delivery quite worthwhile.) Resign yourself to the slightly higher cost as a medical necessity, particularly if you are afraid of falling or if you have heart trouble or arthritis. On the other hand, in good health and good weather a walk to the store for a few groceries is a pleasant way to take exercise and see new faces.

Many older people do not provide themselves with pleasant surroundings and social fellowship at meal times. For company, you might try attending the dinner meetings of senior citizens clubs and church groups in your community. Those who cannot leave their home may make use of a local meals-on-wheels program. The meals are prepared in a central kitchen, usually in a church or in a local hospital, and delivered by volunteers to the participants in their own homes. Often the volunteers bringing the meals provide a social link with the outside world.

Financial strain could mean changes in eating habits and dropping certain foods completely without adding adequate nutritional substitutes. Adequate understanding of nutritional needs and how to meet them in such a situation is of prime importance. The NutriScore rating chart and the foods listed in Appendix A will help you choose less expensive substitutes for food you feel you cannot afford. A balanced diet does not have to be costly.

Older people must have exercise and recreation to accompany the good food. In addition to the limitation of the eating pattern, none of these social, psychological, or financial strains are conducive to encouraging recreation and physical activity, which are particularly important for this age group. Facilities in most neighborhoods are oriented towards youth and are not suitable for older people. This is why communities and villages for retirees are attractive places to live.

We cannot stress enough the importance of being active. You don't have to be an athlete, but you can keep moving at your own speed. Do not overdo it, but never give up devoting time for light sport and recreational activity. Walking is a great habit. Aside from the fact that activity allows you to eat more without gaining weight, it is good for your blood circulation.

The concern older people have for their health can make them easy marks for health food dealers and patent medicine peddlers. This is particularly true with today's aged, who were brought up in an era when one did not go to see a physician until one was almost on the death bed. To them it would seem less costly to accept the claims of health food faddists than to visit a physician. Decisions and attitudes of this type can be very injurious to the health of the individual.

Know your enemy. Understand what the difficulties of aging may be and you have half conquered them. It doesn't make sense to view a change in lifestyle as an admission of weakness. We are changing constantly all our lives, and it's no more shameful for an older person to abandon hearty eating and drinking than it is for a teenager to start consuming double quantities of everything. The results are what count. If cucumbers become indigestible it doesn't matter whether you're pregnant or turning 80; the sensible thing to do is to drop cucumbers from the diet and find their food value elsewhere. At any age our diet affects our physical condition and our physical condition determines our diet.

Consider some of the common hazards of living to a ripe old age: diseases of the heart and arteries can be warded off or their effects minimized by careful attention to the consumption of fat and cholesterol-rich foods, by regular exercise, by smoking less (or preferably not at all), and by eating a well-balanced, modest diet that will keep you healthy and not aggravate tendencies towards diabetes or high blood pressure or other diseases. The best diet in the world will not keep you free from illness, but your diet can make an enormous difference in the effects of illness. Keep your defenses up by eating well at all times.

Osteoporosis is a condition in which the bone and teeth lose calcium and the bones become porous. It leaves its victims subject to easy fractures from the slightest fall.

Osteoporosis results from low supplies of calcium, phosphorus, vitamin D, and fluoride. This means that regardless of how old you are, you never outgrow your need for milk. A glass or two of milk a day will give you all the calcium you need; make sure it is vitamin D fortified. Favor skim milk or two per cent (partly skimmed); they are low in calories and in saturated fat. If you don't like to drink milk, include the equivalent amount in your cooking. Try fish poached in milk or noodles and cheese sauce for main courses. Keep skim milk powder in the cupboard and toss it into mashed potatoes, hot cooked cereal, hamburger patties, and casseroles. If you become accustomed to adding powdered milk at every opportunity you'll find it simpler to meet your daily milk requirements. Remember, one-third cup (75 mL) of skim milk powder is equivalent to one eight-ounce (250 mL) glass of milk.

Loss of teeth for various reasons over the years leaves some elderly people unable to chew all foods. A blender or grater or food chopper can be of great assistance here; don't give up raw carrots before you've tried a grated carrot salad with raisins. And take a new approach. Fresh apples can be served on a plate accompanied by a dessert knife and a wedge of cheese, to give the impression of refined elegance while actually you can cut them small enough to manage with your china choppers. If fresh apples are to hard to chew, baked apples will do. And, pureed vegetables have just returned as the new dining 'chic.'

The flow of saliva is decreased and the sensitivity of the taste buds is reduced as we grow older. Both of these factors result in a change in the taste of food, making it less appealing, and incite old people to add more salt and other flavor substances to their foods. Try the addition of sour and acid substances, such as lemon and lime juice, to foods whenever appropriate. And do experiment with all of the dried herbs on the store shelves. Rosemary is for vegetables, basil for tomatoes, chervil and chives for chicken, and dill seed is good with your fish.

The bile secretions and the digestive enzymes are also decreased and as a result digestion on the whole becomes slightly impaired. This will contribute to a reduction in appetite, to frequent development of signs of indigestion and to constipation. To deal with this situation, chew foods more and eat slowly. More fluids, such as hot soups, and beverages, such as milk, would be nutritious and beneficial in easing the signs of constipation. It might be more convenient and enjoyable to eat frequent small meals rather than a few large ones, and cut down on rich desserts. This will help digestion.

The race isn't run yet, so keep up your supply of fuel. An older man of our acquaintance had a long stay in hospital recovering from a serious operation, and was not tempted (to say the least) by the hospital food. Once home he was catered to by his wife, who soon had him eating everything but vegetables. They seemed distasteful no matter how they were cooked or dressed up, so he simply left them on the plate. However, he was eating and gaining the right amount of weight on the rest of her cooking, so his wife didn't worry until about a year later, when she suddenly saw that her husband hardly had any energy and vitality. Thinking of possible causes, she realized that he must be deficient in some vitamins after a year with no vegetables. A call to the doctor brought agreement with her diagnosis and a prescription for a vitamin and mineral supplement to be started immediately. When that worked, her husband admitted that she knew her business as the household nutritionist, and she eventually got him to eat his peas.

We can't emphasize too strongly the importance of eating daily quantities of fruits and vegetables, whole-grain or enriched cereals and bread, and meat, fish, and eggs. They provide you with protein, and a large variety of vitamins and minerals.

If you have any questions about your diet and whether or not you need a vitamin and mineral supplement, discuss it with your doctor and get a referral to a counselling nutritionist or a dietitian. But whatever you do, do not take the advice of a neighbor, a friend, a health food salesman, or any unqualified person. Rely only on sound medical advice. Everyone in their latter years should be close to a physician to seek advice in a preventive sense and medical care in a curative sense.

REMEMBER

Staying active should be your main concern as you get older and retire. Build activity in the form of recreation and pleasurable sports. You don't have to strain yourself, particularly if you haven't been very active before. But keep going.

Avoid eating alone. As much as possible arrange to share in buying, preparing, and eating food with others.

Keep on testing your diet with the NutriScore chart. Your need for a balanced diet is as great as ever. You may have to drop some of your favorite foods because of chewing or digestive difficulties, but you can pick others from the same area in the NutriScore chart. Never compromise your nutrition.

Don't fall for health fads and medications that promise you youth. It is your continuing activity and interests and your good diet that will sustain your vitality and keep you young at heart.

Nutrition Sense
and
Nonsense

Chapter 15

Sense and Nonsense in Our Food

Here's a chance to double-check your NutriScore. If you marked bread, was it whole grain? Was your rice serving made with parboiled or brown rice? In order to increase your rating, we'd like you to test your sense about the nonsense in some of our foods. Let's find out—what's really in it?

As an old Gilbert and Sullivan song says, "Things are seldom what they seem, skim milk masquerades as cream." There are a lot of false faces confronting the consumer in the supermarket today. Although the government keeps an eye on foods and drugs, they allow at least 300 standard foods, such as mayonnaise, ketchup, and rye bread, to be marketed without an ingredient list. Even when the producer must declare his ingredients, it is left to the customer to interpret the label. Furthermore, much of our food is processed—that is, something has been done to alter its original condition. It is refined, or enriched, or added to, or even manufactured entirely from a chemical formula. To make sense out of this nutritional nonsense, you have to get a firm grip on the terminology, read all labels, and make choices based on sound nutritional guidelines.

Non-dairy creamers are a good case in point. If we are to reduce the amount of saturated fat in our diets, it would be wise to eliminate coconut and palm oil; both these oils are used in coffee creamers, as well as in other products.

Most shoppers are unaware of the degree of saturation of the fat in these "creamers." Others know. One Saturday, for example, Ruth encountered two women, one in her mid-thirties and the other in her late sixties, at the frozen food case. The younger woman reached in and took a container of coffee-whitener and dropped it into her basket while the older woman commented that she could never have that as her doctor had put her on a strict diet that didn't allow her any saturated fats because of her heart condition. She explained that the fat in coffee-whiteners is coconut oil, which is highly saturated. So, why risk it? "Oh, yes," answered the young woman, quite confidently, "I know all about that! But I like the taste!"

Well, no one can argue with that. She obviously knew the facts about the product she was buying; she had knowledge and could weigh the advantages and disadvantages to herself; and she made an informed decision.

If only everyone had the background knowledge.

Since we know that coconut and palm oil are highly saturated, and since we know that manufacturers use them in many mock-dairy products, it is simple to banish foods listing either of these oils on the label—foods such as powdered, frozen, or liquid coffee creamers, whipped toppings, packaged synthetic "whips" and desserts. It would be safer to refuse to use "cream" at restaurants and cafeterias and insist on milk for coffee and tea.

If you must use whipped topping occasionally, why not try whipping evaporated milk. It has much less fat than whipped cream or the substitutes. Be wary of snack foods listing coconut and palm oils on the label. Manufacturers of chips, crackers, cookies, baked goods, and mixes often use coconut and palm oil. They have a pleasant, oily taste on the surface, say the manufacturers; besides which, they are solid at room temperature and don't get youngsters' fingers sticky—hardly a reason to introduce our kids to such saturated fats.

Deciphering the labels is the game. The trick is not to be frightened off by chemical terms, but to learn a few key words that tell how the food has been processed, what is left of the original product, and what has been added. Some words you'll take for warning signals: if they're on the label the package goes back on the shelf. Other terms will induce you to try a different brand, even if you have to pay a few cents more. It's like living by your wits in a foreign land, with only a smattering of the language to help you.

The key words in that label game are: coconut oil, palm oil, hydrogenated vegetable oil. Let's look at some of the others.

"Processed" simply means treated in some way. It is not necessarily a bad word. Some processes, like canning, are beneficial; some, like deep-frying, go too far. The fact is, however, that any processing is bound to destroy some nutrients. Canning and freezing destroy very few, and the benefit of having foods available all year round outweighs these small losses. But when a potato is skinned, steamed, pulverized, combined with chemicals, and deep-fried in fat, very little of the original nutritional content remains.

"Refined": What does it mean? The dictionary says "to purify or separate from extraneous matter." In other words, to take a whole

Nutrients in Boiled and French-fried Potatoes			
	Calories per 100 g	Fat	Starch
Boiled potatoes	65	0.1%	15%
French-fried	275	13 %	36%

food and separate part of it from the rest. This can be as simple as removing the skin from a beet or as extreme as discarding all of the beet except its sugar. Again, every time foodstuffs are refined, some nutritional value is lost.

Why, then, do we refine foods? For taste, texture, appearance, to combine or preserve them, or simply to create a new, competitive product. There are some good reasons for refining. For those who cannot digest whole-grain cereal, it is better to eat a refined cereal than none at all. Unfortunately, many refining processes cater to the consumers' love of fats, sweets, and novelty flavors.

"Enriched". On occasion, foods are enriched, meaning that vitamins and minerals present before refinement are restored or new nutrients are added to improve the nutritional value of the food. Probably, the most commonly enriched food is white flour. To it, the miller adds thiamin, riboflavin, niacin and iron up to the amount that was previously in the grain, but no more. Refinement of flour removes many more vitamins and minerals that are not restored to white flour.

In the United States, calcium is allowed in enriched flour and is usually added. In Canada, calcium is not usually added to flour except in Newfoundland. This province took upon itself to legislate the addition of calcium to bread. They insisted before joining Confederation in 1949 that, because their consumption of milk (the richest common source of calcium) was very low, they should be allowed to legislate the addition of calcium. If ever there was a clear demonstration of the value of supplementation, the present health of Newfoundlanders provides it. Nutrition Canada survey found the diets of the Newfoundlanders higher in calcium than those in other provinces in Canada.

If we want to deal sensibly with our eating habits, we need to look into some of the commonly eaten foods and try to make sense of these familiar products.

Bread can provide all of the nourishment of the whole grain, or it can provide only part of what we could be getting—depending on how far it has been refined. There are some breads that have been made from whole-grain kernels. Not even the wheat germ has been removed and the only nutrient losses have been the ones which inevitably occur in handling and cooking. This is called whole-grain or whole wheat bread and it is the winner.

Cracked wheat bread and white bread rate below the 100 per cent whole wheat bread. Both the bran coat and the germ are removed in making white flour and with them go many of the vitamins and minerals. Most of the fiber, too, is removed along with the bran. This can have unpleasant, and some doctors say serious, effects on digestion and elimination, or lack thereof.

Frozen bread dough is at least as nutritious as fresh bakery bread, and its label must carry a list of the ingredients, so you can look for enriched or whole-grain flour, soya oil, and whatever else you desire. Frozen bread dough is also made without preservatives, an advantage over most store-bought bread.

Some breads are tricky to understand. There is a 60 per cent whole wheat, which the unwary might confuse with the 100 per cent variety. And never equate brown bread with whole wheat. Brown bread is made from white flour, colored with whole wheat flour, graham flour, bran, molasses, or caramel. As for rye bread, only God and the baker know. There are no regulations concerning the proportion of rye that must be present in rye bread. Rye flour, although nutritious, doesn't have strong enough gluten to raise bread, unless combined with white flour.

Enriched white bread does have some vitamins and minerals restored, but it still lacks the pyridoxine, pantothenate, folate, vitamin E, zinc, copper, and manganese present in the whole grain. However, something is better than nothing, so if white bread is going to be part of the regular diet, common sense suggests that

> White bread for the table
> Needs "enriched" upon its label.

Present regulations in Canada make the enrichment of white flour mandatory, but in the United States and many other countries, white flour may be found either enriched or unenriched.

The "New Wave" of the '80s is a return to home baking and cooking. Whether for bread or yogurt, homemakers are streaming to cookery classes in order to regain the natural taste in foods. For home bread baking, the first choice is whole wheat or other whole-grain flours. For more sophisticated loaves, white flour turns out beautiful crisp-crusted French or Italian breads.

Pasta (spaghetti, noodles, macaroni) is made from refined white flour which may or may not be vitamin enriched. In the wide range of pasta products, some are enriched with the B vitamins, thiamin, riboflavin, niacin, and some are not enriched. Enrichment with vitamins is becoming common. Some products have soy flour added to increase their protein level.

If available in your supermarket, enriched pasta with soy added would be our favorite. This type of pasta is regularly available in most "health" food stores. Served with a vegetable sauce, it is a highly nutritious, meatless meal.

Most breakfast cereals are both refined and processed, but some have been man- (or machine-) handled less than others. A few are not refined, like the 100 per cent whole-grain rolled oats and shredded wheat with various brand names. These are labelled as 100 per cent whole grain and contain only the cereal named on the list of ingredients. They are more healthful than cereals made from refined grains. The refined ones are usually diluted with other ingredients. Rolled oats is among the most nutritious of this type because the rolling process does the least damage to nutrients. Shredding is fairly gentle, flaking slightly more destructive, and when those puffed cereals are "shot from a gun," as their ads so proudly proclaim, the extremely high temperature necessary to achieve this remarkable feat shoots much of the good right out of them. So the breakfast table nutritional hierarchy would place rolled oats ahead of shredded whole-grain cereals which precede flaked cereals which are nevertheless above puffed cereals.

Sugar-coating is nonsense. In the first place, it costs more. Compare, for example, the prices of the same brand of Corn Flakes and Sugar Frosted Flakes. The ingredient lists of these two flakes are identical (at least at this writing), *but* the sugared flake has a lot of sugar. If you want to mix sugar and cereal, it's cheaper to do it at home.

In the second place, the sugared flake forces us to eat more sugar than we normally would. Even someone who regularly eats a cereal like Corn Flakes, which already contains a small amount of sugar for flavor, and adds a little more sugar at the table, is unlikely to use as much sugar as the Frosted Flakes contain.

In the third place, so much sugar is downright unhealthy. It programs the tastebuds for sweetness, so that unsweetened foods become unappealing. It fills us up with empty calories, leaving little room for more valuable foods. It rots the teeth. And for some people it raises the risk of heart disease.

Rice is nice and brown is best. But brown rice is not readily available, due to lack of consumer demand. Consumers demand white rice. White or polished rice is a nutritionally denuded product with the vitamins and minerals stripped away when the brown coat and germ are removed. As if this isn't bad enough, manufacturers have developed a product with even greater consumer demand commercially called "instant" or "minute" rice. "Instant" rice is the naked white rice further cooked and dehydrated to avoid 25 minutes cooking time. This removes more nutrients. In our opinion such a sacrifice of nutrients for time is ridiculous. A sensible substitute is the white processed rice known as "parboiled" (or as one manufacturer calls it, "converted") rice. Here is one product in which processing can be said to *add* nutrients.

Brown rice, when parboiled, is steamed under pressure. The pressure pushes many vitamins and minerals from the coat and the germ into the kernel, so that the parboiled rice we subsequently buy has a higher nutritional value than rice kernels naturally possess. Polished rice does not have these added nutrients.

Don't wash rice unless the package specifically tells you to. Most is sufficiently cleaned during processing and further washing may remove some of its water-soluble vitamins.

Freshly dug potatoes which are served immediately retain their full share of nutrients. They contain vitamin C (about 26 mg per 100 g), thiamin, niacin, and iron. After the potato has been six months in storage, thiamin and niacin are decreased slightly, but the vitamin C drops to less than a third (only 8 mg per 100 g).

During preparation, cooking, and holding, the potatoes lose even more, particularly vitamin C. A french fried potato, which is old to begin with, suffers great losses of vitamin C from the slicing, exposure to air, and high temperatures that accompany frying. In addition to the vitamin loss, french fried potatoes have fat clinging to them which increases their fat content. In fact, 70 per cent of their calories are from fat.

Frozen french fried potatoes suffer double jeopardy as they have been peeled, diced, fried, frozen, and then, depending upon which of the package directions you choose to follow for home serving, can be fried *further* or baked. The choices of cooking instructions probably affect iron, thiamin, and niacin very little. Skillet frying or deep frying involve sufficient heating to lower vitamin C. The addition of more fat in the skillet, or deep frying plus the advice to add more salt generously make us cringe! Considering that this is a popular food among adolescents and adults who suffer as a group from obesity, heart disease, and hypertension, such advice is thoughtless, if not irresponsible.

Foods can be synthesized from chemicals, and increasingly they are. Nature puts together many chemicals to make our food. With the current world food shortage and the rise in food prices, we are acquiring and perfecting the technology of combining chemicals to imitate natural food. We are succeeding in making food that tastes, smells, looks, and feels like natural food. But so far the food industry has not been careful to have these fabricated foods contain the same nutritional values as the natural ones they are imitating and replacing in our diet.

It is essential that the nutritional quality of substitute food equals that of the food it is replacing. Several years ago, the Food Service Department in one of our major Toronto hospitals shifted for convenience and economy from orange juice to orange drink (unbeknown to the doctors and the dietitians). It wasn't long before it was noticed that patients in post-surgery were recovering more slowly than expected. One of the dietetic prescriptions after an operation is orange juice, which is given to compensate for the potassium lost during surgery and to provide the patients with the vitamin C needed for healing wounds. The orange "drinks" these patients were getting contained no potassium and the amount of vitamin C was less than that in orange juice, but no one had thought through to the consequences.

The stability of nutrients in substitute foods should also be examined very carefully. For example, vitamin C in orange juice is hardly destroyed at refrigerator temperature. On the other hand, the vitamin C in fruit "drinks" is reduced in quantity when left in the refrigerator for a few days.

Additives—to have or have not? In many of the foods which are formulated in total or in part, chemical additives are introduced to preserve, texturize, color, or flavor the food product. The recommended quantity of these chemical additives has been of concern to government, consumers and industry, and whenever a harmful effect from an additive is demonstrated it is banned. However, sometimes the possible harmful effect of an additive is so subtle that it becomes a subject of speculation among scientists.

For example, many foods such as cola drinks, beer, chocolate drinks, TV dinners and mixes for pizza, cookies, and pastry have phosphates added to them, which is permissible under the food and drug regulations. Phosphates are naturally high in meat and many other foods and are not harmful. In fact, we need phosphorus along with calcium, magnesium, and fluoride to make strong bones and teeth. High intakes of phosphates are not poisonous, *but*, for good nutrition, the ratio of phosphorus to calcium in our foods should be about one to one. So, if we increase phosphorus in the diet we have to increase calcium. Otherwise, we draw calcium from the bones to balance the phosphorus. The main sources of calcium in the diet are milk, cheese, seeds, and vegetables. As long as we are eating many processed foods with phosphates added to them, we have to be particularly careful to take more milk and cheese in our diet. Also, we can just as well avoid cola drinks and other beverages that are particularly high in phosphates.

Some additives look so innocent. Commercially processed foods usually have more salt than we bargain for. Salt contains larger quantities of sodium and excessive intakes are related to high blood pressure or hypertension. Take peas, for example. Fresh or frozen peas contain only 2 mg sodium in a 3 ounce (85 g) serving; the same amount of canned peas contains 236 mg.

Some of the high sodium products include canned and dehydrated soups, canned fish, processed cheese, sausage and processed meats, and nearly all canned vegetables. Many innocent looking foods, such as cereals and puddings, hide a heap of sodium.

It's a wise shopper who makes an informed decision when buying processed foods. Read labels for added salt or sodium in canned, frozen, or packaged products. If possible, always buy fresh and avoid the worry. Of course, it goes without repeating: Go easy on the salt shaker or avoid it altogether.

The Chinese Restaurant Syndrome story illustrates the difficulty additives can cause. Some years back doctors recognized a condition in patients complaining of sudden and sharp headaches, flushes in the head and body, and tingling sensations in the spine. These symptoms eased off and disappeared after a few hours. Over a period of time the patients' case histories made clear one common factor: All ate frequently at Chinese restaurants and the symptoms appeared after such meals. Many of the foods they ate had a chemical called monosodium glutamate (or MSG) added liberally to them. An excess of this chemical was responsible for the patrons' symptoms.

"Accent" is monosodium glutamate, and if we used it as the ads advise, some of us would get Chinese Restaurant Syndrome in our own kitchens. MSG is a natural chemical that is found in every protein and is absorbed readily into the bloodstream, many tissues, and the brain. Since it is readily absorbed in the brain, nutrition scientists identify it among the very few chemicals that cross the brain barrier.

Naturally, there is concern about the wisdom of allowing it in foods. Yet, no one has discouraged its use; in fact, the reverse is true.

"Accent" or MSG is a flavor enhancer, not a necessary ingredient in any food. For the manufacturers to advise consumers to use such a non-essential, risky additive generously is, in our opinion, reckless. Critics of our opinion say that in spite of the reported cases of Chinese Restaurant Syndrome, there is no

Sodium Content of Foods

Food	Size of Serving		Sodium (mg)
Asparagus, fresh cooked	½ cup	(125 mL)	1
Asparagus, canned	½ cup	(125 mL)	185
Bacon, broiled	3 slices	(22 g)	245
Beans, canned with pork	½ cup	(125 mL)	590
Butter, salted	1 pat	(5 g)	40
Cheese, Cheddar	1 oz.	(30 g)	175
Cheese, creamed cottage	½ cup	(125 mL)	455
Cheese, Parmesan	1 oz.	(30 g)	455
Cheese, Roquefort	1 oz.	(30 g)	395
Cheese, processed	1 oz.	(30 g)	405
Cookies, oatmeal	1	(19 g)	35
Doughnut, cake type	1	(32 g)	150
Doughnut, yeast type	1	(32 g)	75
Eggs	1	(50 g)	60
Frozen dinner, meat loaf	11 oz.	(310 g)	1225
Frozen dinner, lasagna	8 oz.	(225 g)	1100
Olives, green	5	(25 g)	465
Pickles, dill	1	(68 g)	965
Popcorn, plain	2 cups	(500 mL)	1
Popcorn, with salt and oil	2 cups	(500 mL)	490
Potato chips	1 cup	(40 g)	400
Salmon steak, broiled	3 oz.	(85 g)	85
Salmon, canned pink	3 oz.	(85 g)	315
Soup, chicken noodle from mix	¾ cup	(175 mL)	610
Soup, tomato canned	¾ cup	(175 mL)	550
Soup, vegetable beef canned	¾ cup	(175 mL)	600
Soy sauce	2 tbsp.	(30 mL)	2665
Tomatoes, raw	1	(150 g)	5
Tomatoes, canned	¾ cup	(175 mL)	230
Tomato juice	¾ cup	(175 mL)	365
Waffles, from mix	1	(64 g)	435

evidence that everyone is susceptible, nor that small amounts of MSG are harmful. Furthermore, it is often argued that deleting MSG from foods would mean their flavor would not be enhanced and people might eat less of them.

The United States National Research Council many years ago convened a scientific panel to assess the situation, specifically with regard to baby foods. Here, there was no argument about babies turning away from foods simply because the flavor is not enhanced. Babies enjoy bland flavors and the longer we delay making their food sweet or salty or meaty, the better eating habits they are likely to develop in later life. The recommendation of the panel was to drop MSG from baby foods, if for no other reason than that it was *not necessary*.

Necessity should be the touchstone for the use of additives. This is an important concept for government to grasp in its regulations and for industry to adopt in its practices. A chemical additive should be not only safe but necessary. Such judgment often requires courage to implement. An example is the addition of nitrites to foods, especially to cured and processed meat. While these additives are not in themselves harmful, they may combine with other chemicals in food or in the intestine to form nitrosamines, which are known to cause cancer. The advantages of using nitrites in processed foods is that they maintain a pinkish-red color, which makes the meat look fresh and attractive, and they check the growth of bacteria. Some of these bacteria, such as botulinum, produce deadly poisons. Government has therefore limited the addition of nitrites to the amount needed to check the growth of botulinum bacteria and no more. Even this small amount may be eliminated altogether as we find a preservative other than nitrite that will be effective against bacteria, yet will not present a cancer hazard.

Cosmetic additives do more than color and flavor our foods. In the early 70s, Dr. B. Feingold suggested that artificial colors and flavors may cause hyperactive behavior in children. This condition, called hyperkenesis, affects some very young children, under 5 years of age, makes them excessively active, inattentive, and readily distractable. It is not a well defined clinical condition, and therefore some physicians either miss it or suspect it incorrectly. Its diagnosis is mainly based on a scoring system developed by Dr. C.K. Conners and known as parent or teacher (P-TQ).

Dr. Feingold's observation excited many parents, teachers, scientists, food industry officials, and politicians. Almost a decade, and many studies and a Senate hearing later, the evidence now points to the notion that it would be prudent to color and flavor our foods *LESS*.

To be sure, there are many studies that give conflicting evidence, mainly because controlled experiments on hyperactivity are not easy to plan or execute. Hyperactive children often benefit from the attention such a study gives them. After all, it takes the teacher's and/or parent's attention to score their condition with Conner's P-TQ. The extra attention helps a great deal. There is evidence that many hyperactive children benefit from a psychological, approach. The study by Dr. Harley and his associates was the largest and best controlled. It involved children over and under 5 years of age. The benefits of an additive-free diet were impressive among the under-5, but not so with the over-5; therefore the findings pointed strongly in favor of dietary management of very young hyperactive children. It is difficult to know not only which colors or flavors affect our children, but how they affect them. Some scientists tend to center their suspicion on artificial colors, particularly an azo dye called tartrazine. But there is little justification to suspect one specific artificial color or flavor over others. Until proven innocent, all should be suspect. Parents, especially of hyperactive children, would do well to manage their own as well as their children's diets wisely. For a dictionary of food additives that may lurk on your kitchen shelves turn to Appendix E: Glossary of Chemicals Commonly Added to Processed Foods.

Are "health foods" a way to avoid over-processing and additives? The trend towards refinement and fabrication of our food supply and the widespread use of chemical additives gave strength to the "health food" movement of a few years ago. There can be no objection to using fresh unadulterated foods in preference to processed or fabricated foods. The truth is that you need to be as careful in shopping at "health" food stores as at any others. An equal number of unsubstantiated claims have been made for the foods sold there, as for the processed foods they seek to replace.

Organic honey, if indeed there is such a thing, is no different in its nutritional value from any other honey. And while honey may contain traces of some vitamins and minerals, it is hardly different from white sugar. The amounts of vitamins and minerals, while adequate for a bee, are so small for humans that we would need to consume enormous quantities to get any benefit.

Granola cereals have the benefit of whole grains but are high in sugar and fat, which make them nutritionally undesirable. A simple home-made granola without dried fruit but with almonds, sesame, and sunflower seeds, oatmeal and shredded coconut, soya flour, wheat germ, powdered milk, honey, and vegetable oil has *146 calories per ounce (30 g), 86 of which (more than half) is fat.* One ounce (30 g) of oatmeal, which makes one cup (250 mL) of cooked cereal, contains *110 calories, of which only 18 calories come from fat.* The amount of protein in both is about the same.

Caveat emptor, "Let the buyer beware," is an ancient saying that is even more relevant today. The manufacturer and storekeeper want primarily to sell. The government wants to protect us while keeping the economy humming. And we want to eat well. All we can do to make sense of these assorted aims is cross our fingers, keep a sharp eye out and think before we eat.

REMEMBER

"Processed" food is not necessarily bad. Over-processing, such as french frying dough for doughnuts or potatoes for french fries, is.

Don't buy products listing primarily coconut or palm oil as ingredients.

Choose whole-grain cereals and breads as often as possible, refined cereals and breads only if they are enriched.

Shun sugar coating. Sugar-coated cereals are over-processed, over-filled with calories, and regrettably low in the balance of nutrients needed for a high NutriScore.

Choose natural foods such as oranges and apples. Substitute foods such as orange and apple "drinks" do not completely substitute for the real thing.

All natural foods are "health" foods. Comparison shop for the best buy, wherever you shop. Don't be hoodwinked by special claims for health.

Additives—let necessity be your guide.

Chapter 16

Confusion in the Supermarket

Shoppers need their wits about them these days. Life would be simplicity itself if a shopping trip meant choices between cabbage or carrots, beef or fish; but today's shopper must race through a bewildering obstacle course of "convenience", "low (or worse still, no) calorie", and "look-alike" products that bear little resemblance to the foods we once knew.

Without losing sight of the fact that cooking and eating food can be joyous, let nutrition be your watchword and NutriScore your guide to easier shopping.

When tripping the light fantastic through the supermarket, keep your balance, start at the produce counter. Vegetables and fruits, fresh, frozen, or canned, should dictate the meals of the week. A well-balanced meal is easy to plan if you take note of the vegetables and fruits in season and build the meals around these. In summer when beans, peas, and corn are plentiful, use chicken, pork, or fish as accents. In winter, choose hearty vegetables such as rutabagas, carrots, and potatoes for beef and lamb meals. Eggs and cheese, beans, and pasta are tributes for all seasons.

The surest test of a good chef is vegetables. Any restaurant where the chef serves pale, limp, soggy vegetables doesn't warrant a return visit. The true food lover treats vegetables tenderly, cooks them, lightly so that the color remains bright and the flavor true, and serves them not as a comes-with to meat, but as a major attraction of the meal.

Choose fresh vegetables when you have a variety and can afford them. Follow the vegetables in season and take advantage of fresh ones in abundance. Don't buy old or wilted vegetables, though. Canned or frozen vegetables are preferable to old vegetables.

When it comes to cooking fresh vegetables, the preservation of nutrients is of prime consideration. Dumping them into gobs of water and cooking the dickens out of them is a disservice not only to the taste, but also the health of everyone.

Fresh vegetables must be washed and sometimes sliced before cooking. When cleaning, be economical. Keep as much of the vegetable as possible. Don't cut the woody stems from broccoli or asparagus; just apply pressure and they will break off at the point where the wood leaves off and the vegetable begins. The less you cut a vegetable, the less chance there is that valuable nutrients will be lost. Green beans should have the ends snapped off and then be cooked whole.

Steaming vegetables is the preferred method because of the short cooking time and low loss of nutrients. An inexpensive steaming basket is one of the best kitchen investments you can make. The vegetable is not immersed in water, the steam cooks it quickly, and none of the nourishment is left to pour down the drain.

While a steaming basket or pot is an excellent investment, you can improvise by using a rack of any kind in a roasting pan; lift it from the water by standing it on Pyrex measuring or custard cups. The Chinese steaming baskets arranged in layers allow you to steam more than one vegetable at a time, saving energy and burner space. Good cooks we know always prepare more steamed vegetables than are needed for a meal. The leftovers are chilled and added to a salad for the next day. Wonderful color!

Steaming Times for Familiar Vegetables

Asparagus spears	10 minutes over simmering water
Green beans	5 minutes over simmering water
Lima beans	15 minutes over simmering water
Broccoli	10 minutes over simmering water
Brussels sprouts	10 minutes over simmering water
Sliced carrots	5 minutes over simmering water
Cauliflower	10 minutes over simmering water
Peas	5 minutes over simmering water
Zucchini	10 minutes over simmering water
Winter squash (½" or 1 cm slices)	15 minutes over simmering water

Just a hint to new mothers: When you begin to prepare foods for baby, remember that steaming saves nutrients, flavor, and time—no messy pot to wash.

To boil vegetables, heat ½ inch (1 cm) of water to boiling in a covered pan and drop the vegetables in just long enough to soften them slightly. To speed up this procedure, use a pressure cooker. Serve and save any leftover liquid for mixed vegetable juice, soup, cooking rice, or reduced and added to any meat or vegetable sauce.

Baking is a nice way to cook vegetables such as squash or eggplant. You can cook a small squash such as acorn or butternut whole; just prick it with a fork to let out the steam, then bake until soft, split, remove the seeds and skin, mash, and season. And potatoes can be baked quickly. If you are in a hurry, just put two metal skewers through the potato and bake it along with the meat loaf, fish, or roast. The metal conducts heat through the potato so that it cooks from the inside as well as out. This cuts cooking time by a quarter or a half depending on the oven temperature. If the oven is on already, you can bake any frozen vegetable in a covered casserole for slightly less than an hour. The best temperature is 325°F (160°C). Simply add one to two teaspoons (5 to 10 mL)of water and a teaspoon (5 mL) of blended butter (see Chapter 4), cover, and bake!

Frozen vegetables should be boiled in the least possible amount of water. Buy the plain vegetables without added sauces, as these sauces add to the cost and dilute the nutrients, besides adding extra fat and seasonings we don't need.

Canned vegetables are nutritious and much cheaper than fresh or frozen at certain times of the year. Long before our noses could reach to the top of the stove, mother used to drain the liquid from canned vegetables and boiled it down slowly in an old aluminum pan. Then she would toss in the peas or corn or whatever just until hot and serve us all of the nourishment she possibly could. We do it to this day, unless there's vegetable soup in the offing, in which case most of the liquid goes into the soup.

The microwave oven is perhaps the most exciting vegetable cooker to arrive on the market as far as we are concerned. Vegetables cooked à la microwave need no water, so all the nutrition stays in until you eat it.

Vitamin C is more bounteous in vegetables than most people imagine, but we must be very careful about the way we shop, store, cook, and preserve them because vitamin C is easily lost. It dissolves in water and is destroyed by heat and by exposure to air.

Potatoes can provide a lot of vitamin C if we handle them properly. A well-organized cook might think it best to pre-prepare dinner early by peeling, slicing and storing potatoes in water for cooking later in the day, so that dinner will be on the table with as little fuss as possible. In fact, vitamin C is lost when the peeled potato is exposed to air; when the cut potato, with even more open surfaces, is dumped into water; and again when the pieces of potato are heated. When a potato loses so much vitamin C over so long a period, very little is left.

Potatoes should be dropped into already boiling water complete with skins, and boiled lightly until just soft. If the potatoes are old, remove the skins and serve. If they are new, brush before cooking to clean off the dirt and serve with a light coating of skin.

Cole slaw is an excellent source of vitamin C. It is made from a rich source, cabbage, and is served raw. But, once the cabbage is grated, it should be used. The vitamin C is easily and quickly oxidized. Day-old cole slaw will have been deprived of much vitamin C. As for the packages of pre-sliced cabbage and the ready-made coleslaw in the supermarket, you can imagine how much vitamin C is left in them by the time they hit your digestive system.

Bring water to the boil before adding the prepared vegetable.

The enzymes that destroy vitamin C when a vegetable is exposed to air are deactivated once the vegetable cooks, so prepare them as the water boils and have them exposed to the air for as short a time as possible.

Don't use baking soda. Granny used baking soda to retain the bright green color of vegetables such as peas, asparagus, and broccoli. Acids and heat turn these chlorophyll pigments a bronzy-green color; we call it army green. Baking soda is alkaline and it used to be thought that it would help retain that fresh green color. Zinc and copper salts act the same way. That's why zinc and copper kettles were often used to make cucumber pickles green. But zinc and copper can form toxic substances during processing and baking soda, while not toxic, destroys vitamin C. Since vitamin C is really more important than the color of the final product, our advice is not to use baking soda when cooking vegetables.

Be very careful when canning vegetables at home. It can be done and it will save money, but not initially, because you positively must buy a pressure canner and use it to process your vegtables. Otherwise, you run the risk of food poisoning, which causes illness, paralysis, and in the case of botulism, death.

Botulism comes from a bacterium that naturally inhabits the soil. When low acid foods are canned without destroying the botulism bacteria, they grow and increase in the food, making it lethal to eat.

Botulism bacteria can be destroyed at high temperatures, but a boiling water bath for however long is not hot enough. Botulism can only be prevented by the maintenance of a high temperature over a long period of time in a pressure canner. This is the method used for commercially canned foods, and it is the only safe method for home canning of vegetables, fish, meat, and the new type of non-acid tomatoes.

Acidic foods such as fruit, sauerkraut, and pickles are not contenders for botulism. Low-acid vegetables such as corn and beans present the most opportunities. Until recently tomatoes contained a lot of acid, but thanks to the development of new strains, you can no longer count on all tomatoes being acidic, so play it safe. Put on the pressure.

Vegetable juices are delightful additions to our diets, mainly for variety and piquant flavor. Vegetable juices are lower in vitamin C and other nutrients than citrus juices, but don't drop them on this account. They add variety, some vitamin C and A, and minerals.

What is that black ring in the can? We have often been asked whether or not the black ring that sometimes forms on an opened can of tomato juice is a sign of spoilage. The answer is no, not really. Each food when canned reacts differently to the various metals in the can so there almost has to be a different "recipe" for each food container. In fact, tin cans aren't just tin. So-called tin cans are actually steel bases with a hundred or more different tin or enamel or other materials lining them according to the product they contain. The important thing is that they are all safe containers.

In the case of tomato products, if you see a black mark where the tomato has come into contact with the cut lid of a tin can, that is really a reaction between the tomato and the base metal which you exposed when you cut through the lid. Since the base metal is steel, this is a reaction with the iron in the metal. We're not suggesting that this is an ideal way to eat more iron in your diet, but none of this discoloration is harmful. Transfer the tomatoes, or other acid foods, to another container if you wish to store them in your refrigerator for a day or two.

If, for any reason, you suspect that the contents of a can have been spoiled, don't taste the food, but throw it away. If you suspect that the food became spoiled before or during processing, save the end of the can with the code number stamped on it and contact your district health authority who can inspect other cans in the same lot, and if necessary, recall a batch. Don't ignore it. Very often, whole lots have been recalled after just such an incident resulting from the observant and quick action of a consumer.

But the brown ring around a ketchup bottle shows there are bacteria present. Once opened, ketchup should be refrigerated. Otherwise, the bacteria that thrive in air and acid (aerobic, acidic bacillus) can grow and multiply. You have probably seen this in restaurants where the ketchup has been kept on the tables without refrigeration. Don't use it at the restaurant and, if it happens at home, remove the brown ring and the ketchup that is exposed to air before you use the balance. From then on, keep ketchup in the refrigerator.

"Eat a salad every day," Grade 1 teachers recite. Salads can excite us in grade 1, but is it any wonder that we learn to tire of them quickly when they are prepared in the same way, day in and day out? The seasons dictate otherwise, but still we persist with some iceberg lettuce combined with flavorless tomatoes doused with repellent orange-colored "French dressing." Anyone who has discovered the secrets of salad making has learned about one of nature's nicest gifts. A salad can be made of any food, and it becomes ambrosia when the combinations are well suited. A happy marriage is spinach and bean sprouts, sliced fresh tomatoes with basil, steamed julienne of turnip and carrot with Roquefort cheese, or dandelion greens tossed with mustard dressing and chopped walnuts. A walk along the produce counter will locate the freshest and the best of vegetables, and a little imagination will provide the rest. If there is nothing fresh, don't panic. Winter or frozen vegetables can be blanched and quickly chilled, then dried with a towel and combined with a light dressing in just the same way as a green salad. Julienned strips of steamed and chilled turnip blend beautifully with blanched, chilled, frozen green beans. Toss with sliced water chestnuts and canned pimiento.

What about salad dressings? Although there are many brands in the supermarkets, a homemade dressing is by far the best choice for salad eaters. When you make your own, you have control over the amount and type of oil. We prefer safflower and sunflower oils as they have a nutty flavor, but some combinations, particularly those with garlic or heavy marinades, cry out for a light olive oil.

A french dressing or sauce vinaigrette should always be freshly made and tossed just before serving with well washed and dried greens. This recipe makes about ½ cup (125 mL)—enough for 6 large salad servings or 8 small ones. This is something the youngest in the family can quickly claim as his specialty!

FRENCH DRESSING—VINAIGRETTE

¼ teaspoon (1 mL) mustard (use English dry or French Dijon prepared)
pinch freshly ground white pepper
6 tablespoons (75 mL) safflower oil
1 tablespoon (15 mL) lemon juice
1 tablespoon (15 mL) red wine vinegar

Place all the ingredients except the oil in a jar or bowl. Mix well. Add the oil gradually, whisking or shaking until well blended. Toss with the salad just before serving. This dressing is fairly bland as it stands and needs some herbs, yogurt, garlic, or cheese to pep it up. Dress it up according to the salad. Dressings for plain salads can be as simple as Vinaigrette or as different as some of these suggested variations.

For chicory, endive, or romaine lettuce: Crush a garlic clove in the salad bowl; add oil, vinegar, salt, pepper and some anchovy paste.

For any salad greens: Rub 2 hard-cooked egg yolks through a fine sieve. Beat in the oil, vinegar, salt, and pepper with a whisk until slightly thickened. Taste and season.

For cabbage or other heavy vegetables: Mix 4 tablespoons (50 mL) of heavy cream with a teaspoon (5 mL) of lemon juice or light vinegar. Taste and add salt and pepper.

For cooked zucchini, potatoes, mixed cooked vegetables: peel and seed 2 tomatoes. Boil them down to half volume, pressing with a wooden spoon; add oil and vinegar. Taste and season with salt and pepper.

For additional flavors to any salad, the most usual garnishes are aromatic herbs, such as chervil, chives, tarragon, and parsley. They are usually coarsely chopped or the leaves are picked and sliced in with the vegetables.

Sliced beet, capers, bread crusts toasted and rubbed with garlic, nasturtium leaves, hard-cooked egg slices, and tomato sections also can be used.

Mayonnaise—a blessing or a curse? Mayonnaise is a creamy, smooth sauce which is prepared by beating oil and egg yolks strenuously until an emulsion is formed. The sauce is made to enhance the flavor of certain foods.

Dill mayonnaise is delicious with cold salmon, tarragon mayonnaise, superb with cooked cold breast of chicken, and so on. With the appearance on the market of prepared mayonnaise and salad dressings, the age-old delicacy of these sauces has disappeared. We now use it for everything, far too often and in too great quantities for both good taste and good health. By its very nature, mayonnaise is high in fat and cholesterol. So make it at home using safflower, sunflower, or corn oil. Mayonnaise does not keep for longer than 10 days in the refrigerator. If you will use less than 1 cup (250 mL), divide the recipe in half (yes, half the egg will do nicely and the other half can be used in scrambled eggs tomorrow). Oh, yes you'll notice there's no salt but our yogurt seasoning trick successfully disguises this. Most mayonnaise recipes call for 2 egg yolks with this amount of oil. Using the blender or food processor method, our recipe contains less egg yolk and therefore lower cholesterol and saturated fat. And, by the way ... on a diet? Dilute the mayonnaise with yogurt, half and half for a nice light taste.

MAYONNAISE

Use a blender or food processor. Makes 1 cup (250 mL)

Ingredients
1 egg
5 teaspoons (25 mL) lemon juice
1 teaspoon (5 mL) dry mustard
¼ teaspoon (1 mL) white pepper
1 cup (250 mL) vegetable or olive oil
2 tablespoons (25 mL) yogurt
herbs of your choice, such as chives, tarragon, chervil, or dill

Method
Combine the egg, lemon juice, mustard, and pepper in the container of the blender or food processor. (If using a food processor, fit it with the steel knife.) Turn on the motor and immediately add 2 tablespoons (25 mL) oil. With the top off and the motor running, add the remaining oil in a thin stream until it is completely used up. Turn off the motor. The mayonnaise should be thick and creamy. If it is too thick, add 1 tablespoon (15 mL) of water. Taste and add the yogurt for flavor and zip. Store mayonnaise in a covered container and refrigerate.

Fresh fruits picked and eaten at their peak are more nourishing than those picked early and shipped or picked at their peak and stored. So, take as much advantage as you can of the fruits in season. We prefer to buy them at our local greengrocer's, because he always has the freshest produce with the least waste. Stopping by at a fruit and vegetable stand every so often is a good way to gauge the freshness of the supermarket produce. You'll also learn quickly what is in season and what is the best buy.

Properly preserved fruit can also provide good nutrition. If you buy produce at its peak and preserve it yourself in the most careful manner, you can be assured of good, nourishing, cheap fruits for the whole year. This is certainly true of home or commercially canned or frozen fruits.

When buying the commercially canned fruits, choose the products with very little or no sugar added. Pick canned fruits with 15 to 20 per cent sugar and less rather than 45 to 50 per cent. Also favor frozen fruits that have been flash frozen and packed without sugar or sugar syrup. These are most often sold in bulk bags without any syrup.

By far the most consistently reliable source of vitamin C throughout the year is citrus fruits, either eaten as fruits, or drunk as a juice.

During certain seasons of the year (especially January and February) citrus fruits are also the cheapest source.

Some time back, publicity was given in the media to a "new theory" that oranges are artificially colored and that this process removes many nutrients. This is illogical and untrue.

As an orange ripens, whether on the tree or in specially created conditions, its vitamin content (and its sweetness) increases to a peak amount when the orange is ripe. Oranges have seasons. During the winter months, they are at their sweetest, juiciest, and fullest. In the summer, or in September and October, when the nights are not cold enough to put the orange color on them, the skins are colored artificially. They are still sweet, juicy, full sized, and just as nourishing. They may be sprayed or treated with ethylene gas for 48 hours to turn the skins orange.

Canned and frozen fruits retain their vitamin C. Since the enzymes that oxidize vitamin C are killed at boiling temperature, canning is quite acceptable for vitamin C rich foods. There are not many of these that are traditionally canned, only strawberries and spinach and various citrus products, but we believe the quality of the nutrients in these canned goods is very high. Freezing is much more popular. Frozen fruits and vegetables and juices can be assessed for their value in the same way as fresh. Our only advice is to stay away from fruits which are frozen with high sugar concentrations. Always buy the fruits in bulk without syrup.

Most of us rely on fruit juices for vitamin C. Some 50 or more juices and drinks on the market today are sold largely for their vitamin C content.

Fruit juice is the natural juice from a fruit to which no water or sugar has been added, unless stated on the label. Natural juice comes as a frozen concentrate to which we add water back to the original volume of the juice; or canned, requiring no dilution. Natural juices contain vitamin C naturally: 64 mg in a 4 oz. (125 mL) glass of orange juice; 46 in grapefruit; 20 in tomato; 11 in pineapple; and 44 in vitaminized apple juice. Apple juice always has vitamin C added and the label will state this together with the amount.

Frozen fruit juices are carefully prepared so that little vitamin C is lost in production. As long as the package is carefully sealed, this vitamin cannot escape. Even if the juice is thawed and refrozen, don't worry. Choose packages that are dry and free of ice crystals on the outside. Ice crystals mean that the package has already been allowed to warm up and then has been refrozen. Fruit juice stains on the packages are a "don't buy" sign. With frozen fruit juice being packed in cardboard containers, splits and breaks are liable to occur. Look carefully before you buy. The freezer thermometer in a supermarket freezer chest should register no more than 0°F (-18°C) and the packages should not be stacked so high that they are allowed to thaw.

If you suspect some thawing has occurred with a frozen juice, you can refreeze it quite safely as long as the juice is still cold and has not warmed to beyond 50°F (10°C). It may tend to separate when you reconstitute it but this is not serious, either for health or nutritional reasons. Refreezing can change the texture, appearance, and flavor, but the food value remains. Food poisoning micro-organisms would have difficulty growing in a naturally acid medium such as citrus juice. We certainly do not recommend careless handling of any food product; however, the odd softening of a frozen juice carton, as long as it has not split, does not constitute a threat to health.

Fruit drinks are not natural juices although some contain some natural juice and some natural flavor. Don't be misled by such statements on the label as "Drink made from freshly squeezed oranges." The operative word here is drink. The listing of fresh orange juice among the ingredients should not distract you from noticing that other ingredients have been added. Although many drinks contain juice concentrate or pulp, there are those that do not contain any part of the fruit. For example, one brand lists sucrose, dextrose syrup, orange pulp, citric acid, vegetable oil, gum arabic, cellulose gum, sodium nitrate, calcium, phosphate, artificial and natural flavor. You could hardly equate that with orange juice.

Fruit drinks are enriched with vitamin C. But there are many other nutrients naturally present in the juice that are not added. In the case of orange juice, there are significant amounts of potassium, iron, and thiamin. And the vitamin C protectors that occur naturally in orange juice are not present in orange drinks. This means the vitamin C in drinks, while present in the factory, vanishes from the opened pitcher or can at home.

This is not so with natural orange or grapefruit juice, either frozen or canned. A recent study compared the stability in fresh, frozen, and canned orange juice. The juices were prepared for consumption and stored at room temperature or in the refrigerator in closed glass containers. Even after eight days, the vitamin C content was essentially unchanged, regardless of storage temperature.

Pause for a while at the dried beans, peas, and lentils, as you thread your way through the aisles of the supermarket. Because they are low fat, highly nutritious store houses, with high protein content, rich in thiamin, riboflavin, iron and other minerals, home cooked beans and lentils are gaining favor, especially as food prices rise. Most of these dried legumes are available in plastic bags well labelled as to their content and weight. When buying them remember that they cook to double their size. They keep cooked in the refrigerator for one week and in the freezer for one month. But we recommend that you cook only as much as you'll need for the day and keep the balance dry in a covered jar.

The cooks of our generation can well remember Granny's methods of preparation; for us, it is simple to whip up a bean soup or stew. Younger people, however, who would like to buy and cook these products do not know where to look for information. The cook books of today either don't include the basics or, when they do, the suggestion is to use the canned or processed variety of bean. That is hardly necessary, for bean cookery is simple. Cost is not the only reason for using dried legumes, lentils, and beans. If humanity is to survive, our own protein and calorie needs will increasingly have to come from vegetable sources. Red, white, and kidney beans, black-eyed peas, and lentils are the "plain janes" of the kitchen, just ready and waiting to be transformed into the "fair ladies" of the dining room.

Red kidney beans are shaped like a kidney. They are simple to cook and store, and we use them hot for chili con carne with cornmeal pancakes or cold for salads.

White beans are round and white, often favored for baked beans or soups.

White pea beans are similar to white beans, although oval, traditionally used as baked beans.

Lentils are indispensable to a thick marrow bone soup. They are tiny and usually sold split. Cook them quite quickly and add to a soup (along with the liquid) or toss in with rice or bulgar wheat for a side vegetable on a meatless night.

Dry peas can be bought, either split for split pea soup, or whole for a vegetable combination dish with rice or barley. The whole peas should be soaked and cooked as beans. The split peas are quicker cooking for soup.

Chick peas (garbanzo beans) are white, relatively large (compared with dried peas), and can be used in soups, or stews, blended with sesame for a spread, or cooked and eaten cold as a snack. They are delicious in a tossed salad.

Black-eyed peas are traditionally a specialty of the southern United States. These peas are small and white with a black spot on one side. They are indigenous to "soul food" and delicious with rice and tomatoes and homemade bread.

Black beans are small and black. They are often stewed and served hot and spicy, with red and green peppers offering the "bite" to the dish.

Soybeans are the miracle workers of the bean family. While all beans and peas give you 4 g to 5 g of protein in a serving of one cup of cooked beans, soybeans give 10 g of protein in the same size serving. They can be served as a bean, much as any other, or used as soy grits to add texture to a mixed vegetable dish.

They are the basic ingredient of textured protein products which are sold in three ways: as look-alikes for some meat products; as meat stretchers; and as a combined meat and soy product.

Historically, baked beans have always been served with brown bread, and lentil stew with rice, just as chili was traditionally served with cornmeal. Tradition is something to be remembered, even when cooking.

A good proportion of cereal products taken in combination with the beans will reduce the flatulence often associated with them. Each person's tolerance for beans is quite unique, but serving more or less bread, rice, corn, or other cereal grain or vegetables should help. Just experiment until you find your own level of tolerance.

Peanut butter, the spread made from pulverized peanuts, is a good food, especially for children and growing teens. It supplies protein, carbohydrates, and a vegetable source of fat, all of which are needed by a youngster for growth and energy.

Spread peanut butter lightly on toast in the morning in place of butter. Combined with bread and a glass of milk this is a protein-rich meal. But remember that 1 tablespoon (15 mL) equals 100 calories, so "lightly" is the word.

Almost all peanut butters in supermarkets are homogenized and have hydrogenated oil or a monoglyceride added. Homogenization and hydrogenation are two entirely different procedures, but in the processing of peanut butter, they generally occur together. Homogenization makes the mixture smooth, and the addition of hydrogenated peanut oil keeps it smooth and prevents the oil from going to the top. Homogenization is a physical (not chemical) process that reduces the size of the fat globules to form a smooth emulsion. It mechanically disperses the oil, but does not alter the chemistry. Hydrogenation, on the other hand, is a chemical process that adds hydrogen to the oil and makes it more saturated.

It is possible to buy and make natural peanut butter. Natural is the way all peanut butter used to be, before somebody realized that people would pay to have the oil stirred in for them. You can buy plain peanut butter that is not only unhomogenized and unhydrogenated but also has no added sugar or salt as many peanut butters do, at "health" food stores and sometimes in large supermarkets.

The peanut butter to avoid is the one with added hydrogenated oil, sugar, salt, or jams and jellies. There is no excuse for a manufacturer to clutter a simple product such as peanut butter with ingredients that play on the weaknesses of children for a sweet taste and a smooth texture while increasing their health risks.

Cereal is the first solid food to pass our lips as infants and the starter for each new day thereafter. It is an important part of the diet. Everybody talks about it and almost every manufacturer is doing something to it. Too much, in our opinion. Don't let all the ballyhoo befuddle you. The best nutritional and economical value still comes from unrefined hot cereal; next to that is the refined cereal with vitamins and a little or no sugar added. Never forget that the Scots withstood inclement climate, inhospitable terrain, and Imperial England, thanks in part to their penchant for nourishing hot oatmeal.

Hot whole-grain cereals are best not because they are hot (although there's something about a steaming pot of fragrant oatmeal on a cold morning), but because they are unrefined and only slightly processed. Although you should be aware that a few refined hot cereals such as Cream of Wheat, and unrefined hot cereals, such as corn meal, are not as nourishing as wheat, rye, or oats. Ready-to-cook whole-grain cereals are the best choice at the cereal counter. There are plenty of them to choose from. Most grocery shelves carry a selection of wheat, oats, flax, and other seeds for nourishing hot cereals. And then, of course, there are the oatmeals.

"Instant" oatmeal, although it tastes like any other hot cereal, has been steam-treated, rolled, then cooked and dried, and this processing can affect any of the water-soluble or heat-sensitive nutrients. It also frequently contains added salt used to gelatinize the starch and reduce cooking time, and is, therefore, not suitable for anyone on a salt-reduced diet.

"Quick" oatmeal has been processed too, although not as severely. Despite the nutrients lost by subjecting it to heat, it still contains more food value than any cold cereal.

Regular oatmeal is made from hulled and rolled oats and scotch-type oatmeal from oats that have merely been ground. Most of the nutrients and fiber remain for our benefit. They are not hard to cook. And washing the pot afterwards will be no problem if you soak it in cold water. Should your package direct you to add the oatmeal to boiling water and then cook for one hour in a double boiler or for 20 minutes over direct heat, don't give up in despair. We have found you can start water boiling over direct heat in both parts of the double boiler, add oatmeal to the top section, put top over bottom, cover, set the table and pour the juice, and serve in 20 minutes. (Use 3 cups (750 mL) of boiling water to 1 cup (250 mL) of raw oatmeal.) If you have a microwave oven the oatmeal goes in a bowl with water or milk and cooks in less than a minute. With any method toss in a handful of raisins with the oatmeal and eliminate the need for sugar.

The main thing about unrefined hot cereals is that they contain most of the vitamins, minerals, and protein of the wholesome grains they are made from. Some cold cereal manufacturers claim to have added missing vitamins and minerals back to refined grains, but the truth is they haven't added all of them. In Canada, the manufacturers are allowed to add only three vitamins (thiamin, riboflavin and niacin) and one mineral (iron). In the United States, although more vitamins and minerals are added, the list doesn't include many of the trace elements that are needed by the body. Also, fiber is not added. So, the enriched refined cereal is never as good nutritionally as the wholesome unrefined cereal. Also, a bowl of refined cold cereal because of so much processing, costs at least 50 per cent more than, and often three times as much as a bowl of unrefined hot porridge.

Cold cereals deserve their innings, however. We need them for variety, for an early start on camping trips and for smoldering hot days when we can't face hot cereal.

Enriched cereals are not the simple solution their makers would have you believe. We have to ask ourselves: Do we need what they offer, will we really get it, does an undesirable sweetener come along with it, and are we paying a lot more money for very little more nourishment?

Iron, for example, is added back to most refined cereals, but it is doubtful whether all of the added iron is in a form that the body can use efficiently. The form of iron in iron pyrophosphate cannot be used as completely by the body as in ferrus sulfate. Coarse reduced iron is not used by the body as well as the fine-meshed grades (10 microns or less). Read the label; if you have a choice, pick the cereals enriched with ferric sulfate or reduced iron in preference to those containing iron pyrophosphate.

Since milk is supposedly always added to cereals, it can be argued that what you lack in the refined cereal you will get from the milk. This argument is often used by manufacturers with particular reference to protein, but it is irrelevant. You see, cereals should be as nourishing as the grains from which they are made; no less, no more. The fact that they are eaten with milk does not justify processing much of the nourishment out of them.

When it comes to protein we need to think not only of the amount of protein, but also of the nutritional quality. For example, an ounce of Special K has more protein than an ounce of rolled oats. But, the quality of protein in rolled oats is much higher and compensates for the slightly lower protein level. In the U.S. a manufacturer can claim high protein on the basis of the amount in the product, while in Canada any

Per cent of Daily Protein Allowance of an 8-Year Old

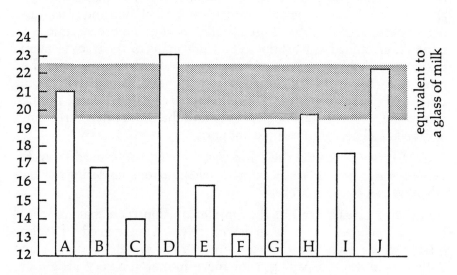

A 8-oz. (250 mL) milk
B 1-oz. (30 g) corn flake + 4-oz. (125 mL) milk
C 1-oz. (30 g) puffed corn + 4-oz. (125 mL) milk
D 1-oz. (30 g) oatmeal + 4-oz. (125 mL) milk
E 1-oz. (30 g) cream of rice + 4-oz. (125 mL) milk
F 1-oz. (30 g) puffed rice + 4-oz. (125 mL) milk
G 1-oz. (30 g) cream of wheat + 4-oz. (125 mL) milk
H 1-oz. (30 g) shredded wheat + 4-oz. (125 mL) milk
I 1-oz. (30 g) puffed wheat + 4-oz. (125 mL) milk
J 1-oz. (30 g) high protein flake + 4-oz. (125 mL) milk

Source: Womack, M., Vaughan, D.A. and Miller, L.R., J. *Food Science 39:* 371, 1974

claims for the value of protein in a food are based on a rating that combines the amount and the nutritional quality of protein. Cereal manufacturers get around the regulations in Canada by claiming for the rating of the combination of the cereal and the milk. Thus, you'll notice the statement on boxes of these cereals, "One ounce of this cereal taken with four ounces of milk is a good dietary source of protein." This is misleading to consumers. Make no mistake about it; a regular glass of milk is in itself a good dietary source of protein. As consumer author Sidney Margolius puts it, "If milk is the main nutritional value in eating dry cereals, then obviously there are easier ways to drink it than with a spoon." To illustrate this point, the graph opposite compares the value (quantity and quality) of a variety of cereals plus milk with that of a glass of milk alone. There are few that can claim to be equal to or better than a glass of milk.

Sugar-coated cereals are the bane of the nutritionists' existence. Not only are they a wasted item at mealtime, but all too often they are used as snacks that will diminish the appetite for proper meals.

On no other shelf in the food market will you find so many products heavily coated and deep-heat treated with so much sugar as on the cereal shelf. On no other shelf will you pay so much for sugar, either.

Ingredients must be listed on labels and in advertising showing the largest amount first and thereon to the smallest amount. In many "cereals" that are heavily sugared, sugar appears at the top of the list or very close to the top. Even in some "health" cereals, sugar is close to the top of the list. It may be called honey, or dextrose or glucose, but the effect is the same—more sugar than we need for more than we should pay!

Granola is a cereal that seems to have originated from a traditional Swiss recipe. Basically, it's a heat-treated combination of grains, honey, skim milk powder, shredded coconut, seeds, and nuts.

We spent some time evaluating the nutritive value and cost of home recipes. We then compared the nutrients in a one-ounce (30 g) serving of granola with the same amount of Special K, unenriched Corn Flakes, and oatmeal. We found about one and a half times more calories in granola, due mainly to the fat content of seeds, nuts, and wheat germ. True, granola needs no further sweetener but, even when we added one teaspoon (5 mL-14 calories) of sugar to the other cereals, granola still had appreciably more calories. Granola is higher in protein than Corn Flakes, about the same as oatmeal, containing approximately a third less than Special K. Granola has a very much higher calcium content (five times the amount found in oatmeal or Special K) because of the skim milk powder and sesame seeds.

Our conclusion was that granola does have *slightly* more protein, calcium, riboflavin, and niacin than plain cereals, but the difference is not great enough to make this a special reason for buying it. Its major disadvantages are its high caloric value, its high fat content, the high saturation of fat in the shredded coconut, and its high cost.

If you wish to purchase commercially prepared granola cereal or "health" cereals, be sure to check the label first. In some products you will find sugar high on the list of ingredients, and there may also be too much fat content from nuts, seeds, coconut, and added oils.

In the dairy case you will find a variety of nourishing foods. But even there, you will have to learn to choose wisely.

Whole milk can contain from 3.0 to 3.25 per cent fat. Our friends are often surprised to learn that whole milk has only about 3 per cent butterfat. That small number is deceiving, because in terms of calories, that 3 per cent fat is really 50 per cent of the calories from fat. A glass of milk is 160 calories, of which 80 calories are from fat.

Most of the fluid whole milk marketed and all of the fluid partially skimmed milk are homogenized. This involves pumping pasteurized milk under pressure through very small openings, breaking up the fat into minute globules that are immediately surrounded by a film of protein that prevents them from re-uniting.

The 2 per cent milk is simply milk with 2 per cent milk fat rather than 3.5 per cent. If your family likes a little fat with their milk, 2 per cent milk is better than whole milk although the calories in an 8-ounce (250 mL) glass are still high—140 compared with 86 in a glass of skim milk. It would be far better to lower the calories by mixing 2 per cent milk with skim or reconstituted skim milk.

Skim milk has had almost all the fat removed. According to food and drug regulations, the fat content of skim milk cannot be higher than 0.1 per cent.

Filled milk is a skimmed milk product which has a vegetable oil added to bring the taste closer to that of whole milk. The argument in its favor is that vegetable oil lowers the cost of the milk and reduces the amount of animal fat.

Filled milk of various kinds began appearing in the United States in the late 1960s. These milks are allowed in some states depending on the state laws. Filled milk has not made its appearance in Canada because of a rather restrictive federal law.

Is filled milk an adequate nutritional substitute for whole milk? It remains to be proved. The only nutritionally significant difference between filled milk and whole milk is the type of fat used. Some manufacturers have used coconut oil because of its desirable taste and physical properties. This has its dangers if given to babies or to persons on modified-fat diets. Coconut oil is low in essential fatty acids and polyunsaturates and therefore would not meet the requirements of such a therapeutic diet.

As much as we favor the use of a properly formulated filled milk, our strong belief is that its formulation and the claims made for it should be carefully regulated. U.S. consumers can be misled into believing that a filled milk advertised as containing only 1 per cent butterfat is lower in calories than regular whole milk. In fact, it is not. Only the type of fat has been changed to lower the cost.

A properly formulated filled milk containing a polyunsaturated fat would close a noticeable gap in the overall nutritional quality of dairy foods. But we still very much favor the use of skim milk at all times—either in liquid or powdered form.

Skim milk powder has so much going for it, it's surprising that it hasn't caught on more. It is cheaper than fluid skim or whole milk.

Skim milk powder saves calories from fat. Fifty per cent of the calories in whole milk is from fat; the percentage of calories from fat in skim milk is zero.

In addition, most dried milk processors are now fortifying their skim milk powder with both vitamin A and vitamin D. The vitamin A that occurs naturally in milk is lost when the fat is removed, so a water soluble form of vitamin A is added. Vitamin D does not naturally occur in milk or in any of our foods in large enough amounts to be useful, so our only sources are vitamin D enriched foods or vitamin preparations. Vitamin D is added to milk in a water soluble form. Its addition to milk was promoted in Canada in the late 1960s in response to medical reports of a high incidence of rickets in children. The startling decline of this disease since then shows that vitamin D diet enrichment is working!

We've heard all sorts of objections to skim powder. The two we hear most often are "it tastes artificial" and "it doesn't dissolve well." As to the first—the processes used today have resulted in a product that tastes much more like fluid milk, and, you'll find that it tastes better when it is made up several hours ahead of time and stored in the refrigerator. When it is icy cold, the flavor has a chance to mellow. If your family still doesn't like the taste, mix it half and half with fluid milk. As the weeks go by you can increase the amount of reconstituted milk and decrease the amount of fluid milk.

"Milk powder doesn't dissolve in water." Today's instantized versions aren't a problem. The milk has been dried, moistened with steam, and then redried (or instantized), and it combines rapidly when added to water. If the milk powder goes lumpy, either buy it in smaller quantity or store it in the refrigerator. Don't leave the top open, because the powder absorbs moisture from the air, causing lumps.

Milk powder has a few other advantages. You can store far more of it in a smaller space than fresh milk. (Our families drink so much milk that the refrigerators would be cluttered with three-quart jugs.) Skim milk powder makes a whipped topping that can be used in place of cream. You can add extra powder to cakes and cookies, too. If you're looking for a place in your food budget to save money, skim milk powder will give the same nutrition for about a quarter the price.

Buttermilk is smooth and tangy, so much so that you'd imagine it to be milk with fat added and very high in calories. It isn't; rather, it is a pasteurized skim milk fortified with skim milk solids to which an acid culture has been added. If the flavor is too strong for you, mix it with fluid or reconstituted skim milk to suit your taste.

Yogurt is a fermented milk food, made from partially skimmed milk, or sometimes whole milk, and bacterial cultures which give it a custard-like consistency without the cloying sweetness of a custard dessert. It is much more popular than buttermilk, although both have the same characteristic taste and nutritional value. Yogurt is more expensive than milk, but it makes such a good dessert that it is worth including in your diet.

Commercial yogurt is made from fresh, fluid, partially skimmed milk that has been pasteurized, then bacterial culture added. Then for several hours the temperature is carefully controlled. During that time the acidity is also checked so that the flavor of different batches will always be the same. When it is tart enough, it is cooled immediately to 40°F (5°C). Fruit or flavoring is added. The regular style yogurt contains a bit of gelatin to make it firm. The Swiss-style yogurt is less solid and has a higher butterfat content that makes it creamier.

The calorie count varies from brand and brand and from flavor to flavor. A half cup (125 mL) of plain yogurt has 65 to 100 calories. The fruit-flavored yogurt is much higher in calories, 115 to 165 in that same half cup (125 mL).

There are many commercial varieties of yogurt on the market today. Some are pure milk with added bacterial culture. Some have other chemicals added to stabilize, emulsify, and lengthen shelf life. So the labels of some will list such ingredients as potassium sorbate, gelatin, corn starch, carageenan, and pectin. If a commercial yogurt is made properly, chilled, and transported and stored with care, none of these is necessary. We would rather walk an extra block for a pure milk yogurt than settle for one with all these additives. After all, if the yogurt is fresh and cold, why put them in, and if it isn't, do we really want to eat it?

Making yogurt at home can save you money. It is a fairly simple procedure. Start with a tablespoon of commercial natural yogurt (not the type with gelatin or gums) to act as a culture and save a tablespoon each time to start a new batch. Add this yogurt to boiled, lukewarm milk and let it sit in a warm place for several hours to thicken. The temperature of the milk must be exactly right when you add the yogurt culture or it won't thicken. Making yogurt is similar to making a yeast bread or junket dessert—too hot a temperature will kill the culture, too cold a temperature will prevent the culture from growing.

With a little experimenting you can make yogurt to suit your taste—thick or thin, tart or bland. Add your own favorite flavoring or fruit, but don't forget to save some plain yogurt to use as a culture for the next time.

Cheese is an excellent food that combines many of the nutritional qualities of milk with a chewy texture and any one of a variety of sophisticated flavors. Some cheeses, such as Mozzarella, are relatively bland (good for sauces on a pizza or lasagna), while others, such as blue cheese, are flavorful by themselves or on a cracker. There are hard cheeses to slice or grate and soft ones to spoon out or spread.

Harder cheese can be kept in the refrigerator for longer than soft cheeses. Wrap any cheese in moisture-proof wrapping and it will keep for several weeks. Some cheeses—Cheddar, Swiss, edam, and gouda—can be stored in the freezer if frozen quickly in small packages (½ lb. or 225 g); however, it is best to avoid having so much cheese that you have to freeze it, as there is some deterioration in quality and texture.

All cheeses are high in protein. In cheese making, the protein from milk is curdled. But there are rich high fat cheeses made from milk and cream; some, which are low in fat, are made from skim milk or partly skimmed milk.

Low-fat cheeses are hard to come by, but a variety are on the market if you search. They are not as smooth and rich-tasting as the ones made from whole milk. Some people have an instant dislike for skim milk cheese and so the cheeses made with partly skimmed milk offer a palatable compromise. They are lower in fat than ordinary cheeses but have a better flavor and texture than those made with pure skimmed milk.

Cottage cheese is a low-fat cheese. It is made by cooking pasteurized skim milk, evaporated skim milk, or skim milk powder until it separates into curds and whey. The enzyme, rennet, and lactic acid are used to help form and set the curds. The whey is drained off and the curds washed. Dry cottage cheese is packaged and sent to the grocery store with no extra handling.

To creamed cottage cheese, a dressing is added to the curds after washing. The dressing contains cream (about 2 tbsp. (25 mL) of table cream for every 8 oz. (225 g) cottage cheese). A bacterial culture of harmless acid-producing bacteria, salt, sometimes skim milk powder, an emulsifier, and a preservative such as potassium sorbate or sorbic acid are added; some calcium chloride also may be added. A fruit or relish will produce a fancier variety.

Creamed cottage cheese must contain a minimum of 4 per cent butterfat and each ½ cup (125 mL) serving has 130 calories. The dry cottage cheese has about 90 calories for that same ½ cup (125 mL). For the calorie-conscious person, there are some low calorie "creamed" cottage cheeses on the market. But you can save calories by simply draining the creamed cottage cheese. This will remove some of the cream and some of the calories, too.

Creamed cottage cheese does not have as long a shelf life as the dry variety because it contains cream, and because it requires extra handling when the dressing is added. However, it should keep for at least a week. Dry cottage cheese should keep for up to three weeks. Check the date on the package when you buy it.

If you're really calorie-conscious and want to use dry cottage cheese, you can make it more flavorful by adding seasonings such as onion salt, parsley, chives or even a little milk to make it more moist.

Cottage cheese, even the creamed version, is an economical source of protein and is low in calories. It has less calcium than other cheeses, but it is still an excellent dairy food.

Processed cheeses are made from natural cheese, emulsified and stabilized and extruded into different shapes to become cheese spreads, slices, or other processed cheese food. Natural cheeses, such as Cheddar or Camembert cheese, develop flavor with age. Flavor is as much a part of a good aged cheese as taste and texture. In processed cheeses the aging is stopped before they have a chance to ripen and in our opinion they lose personality when this is done. In addition, a color and a preservative such as propionate or sorbate are added to processed cheese to prevent bacteria and mold from growing on it. Boring as we consider the result, this cheese does have the same nutritional value as natural cheese.

The availability of processed cheese in different forms makes it a versatile product that may be used in many foods. Skim processed cheeses are preferable to whole-fat processed cheeses because their fat content is lower. As for taste, the tanginess of a natural cheese is a treat that mustn't become a thing of the past. Considering the rate at which processed cheeses sell, however, it seems possible that many of today's youngsters will grow up without any appreciation of the taste of real cheese!

Cream cheese is very high in fat and should be left out of the diet most of the time. Ninety-one per cent of its calories come from fat.

It's easy and tasty to substitute cottage cheese for cream cheese. Add a dollop of yogurt to make a sandwich spread, or make a cheese cake. Here is a recipe you might like to try.

CHEESE CAKE

Crust
⅔ cup (150 mL) crushed graham wafers
3 tbsp. (50 mL) finely chopped pecans
1 tbsp. (15 mL) wheat germ
¼ tsp. (1 mL) cinnamon
1 tbsp. (15 mL) skim milk powder
2 tbsp. (25 mL) Blended Butter (Chapter 4)
Combine ingredients and press into an 8" springform pan. The recipe may be doubled for a larger sized springform pan. Set aside for filling.

Filling
2 egg whites
1 whole egg
1 lb. (500 g) 2% fat cottage cheese
1 tbsp. (15 mL) corn starch
*¾ cup (175 mL) sugar
1 tsp. (5 mL) vanilla extract
1 tsp. (5 mL) lemon extract
½ cup (125 mL) yogurt
Combine all ingredients, except yogurt, in large blender jar. Blend for 1 minute or until ingredients are blended smoothly. Pour into crust and bake at 375°F. (190°C) for 10 minutes. Lower oven temperature to 225° F (120°C) and continue baking for 1 hour. At 45 minutes of final baking time, open oven and spread yogurt over cake. When time is up turn off heat and leave cake until oven is cool. Refrigerate. Cut into 1" (3 cm) squares. Serves 8-10. Cake can be topped with fresh fruit or fresh fruit glazed with gelatin.

*Some or all sugar may be replaced with non-nutritive sweeteners, such as saccharin; taste as you add.

Ice cream, soft ice cream, ice milk, or sherbet? These products are all different, but relatively few of us can distinguish between them, and many of us wonder which are "healthiest" for our families, particularly for the junior set.

Ice cream or soft ice cream cones are a delightful (and quite acceptable) treat for the children. But "treat" they should be, *not* regular fare. Ice cream has the nutrients of milk, but with many more calories. One cup of ice cream has the nutrients of ½ cup (125 mL) of milk, but four times the calories. And adults are reminded that the calories originate, in large measure as fat. So, our advice to grownups is that ice milk or sherbet are the best choice on a hot Sunday afternoon. Don't consider them a regular dinner-time dessert.

Regular ice cream contains at least 10 per cent milk fat (the deluxe products have even more). It is made from a pasteurized combination of cream, milk, or other milk products, plus sugar, invert sugar, honey, dextrose, glucose, and corn syrup. It may contain egg, a flavoring preparation, a stabilizing agent, and a sequestering agent. The whole mix is frozen and then whipped until it has doubled in volume.

Soft ice cream is similar; it has the same milk fat, slightly more solids and less sugar than ice cream. It is whipped to be only one and a half times its original volume. The finished product is equally as rich as hard ice cream.

Mellorine is a soft ice cream product, made with hydrogenated vegetable oil to replace the animal fat, just as in hard margarine, coffee creamers, and filled milk, made with coconut oil. These products are not for you.

Ice milk contains less fat (3 per cent compared to 10 per cent) but more sugar than ice cream. It is a saving in calories—but still quite rich.

Dietetic ice cream-type products are available, but they are not for dieters; they are for carbohydrate-restricted diets. Made with artificial sweeteners and "recommended for sugar reduced diets", they have a 6 per cent fat content and 140 calories per ½ cup (125 mL) and are not as good a nutritional bargain as ice milk.

Calories Chart

½ cup (125 mL) regular ice cream	—160 calories
½ cup (125 mL) premium ice cream	—190 calories
½ cup (125 mL) ice milk	—130 calories
½ cup (125 mL) soft ice cream	—160 calories
½ cup (125 mL) dietetic ice cream	—140 calories

Why not make it yourself? Recipes for homemade ice cream come out every summer like the groundhog in February. They are circulated and tried by everyone, much to the eater's delight. For the enjoyment they bring, sherbet or low-fat iced desserts are popular with sophisticated diners and well worth the time spent in preparation. We particularly recommend the apricot, fresh raspberry, and strawberry sherbets in volume two of Julia Child's *Mastering the Art of French Cooking*.

For low-calorie hot weather desserts, try the ones in the *American Heart Association Cookbook:* champagne ice, ginger ale sherbet, and lemon sherbet. These are all pretty glamorous and not intended as handouts at juice-and-cookie-time during summer school break.

For children, try freezing yogurt as popsicles—tangy, delicious and nourishing! Or prepare milk puddings and freeze them—or freeze fruit juices for a very hot day when a crowd of little people assault your kitchen. You'll be surprised at the savings in cost. And there is the security of knowing that the children are enjoying natural, nourishing, and reduced-fat desserts and snacks.

Ice cream keeps well in a freezer (0°F or -20°C or lower) for one month. Homemade ice cream should be fast frozen at -10°F. (-25°C); packaged in freezer containers; it can be stored for one to two months. Always cover the cut surfaces with waxed paper.

What about eggs? Should we? Shouldn't we? Unless your doctor eliminates them from your diet, never drop eggs completely from your shopping list. Moderation should be your motto. Allow yourself three to seven eggs per week. For those over the age of 40, try to live with three or four eggs a week—no more and no fewer.

Eggs are far too valuable nutritionally (containing protein, iron and other minerals, vitamin A, thiamin, riboflavin, and other vitamins) to have fewer than three a week. A person whose blood cholesterol is high is usually advised by his doctor to stay away from foods heavy in cholesterol and fats, such as eggs. But a doctor should also ensure that his patient's nutrient needs are met in other ways. For the rest of us, three eggs a week are essential, and if we are below the age of 40 and in good health, slim and fit, we can have as many as seven.

How do we cook our eggs? The case for egg yolk! Boiling and poaching are perfect ways to cook an egg. But eggs are protein and any protein food should be cooked gently. Keep the water simmering, not boiling, and add a teaspoon (5 mL) of vinegar to the water for poaching in a covered flat pan so that the white will congeal quickly to a perfect flat shape.

We've been asked about the egg yolk that is left after making blended butter and the answer, aside from making custard sauce, adding it to meat loaf, as a coating for French Toast, baking cookies or adding to shampoo as an egg shampoo, is to scramble it. For two servings, add one tablespoon (15 mL) water to one egg and one yolk (always treat the yolk as an egg for the purpose of your weekly intake calculation) and beat well with a whisk. Preheat pan, brush lightly with oil, (or use special oil-less pan), add mixture and stir over low-medium heat until congealed. Add pepper after cooking; it toughens an egg if you sprinkle it on first.

Another approach is to add skim milk powder. In our experience, however, milk tends to toughen eggs. If this has not been your experience, add one or two tablespoons (15 mL) of powdered milk and one tablespoon (15 mL) of water before whipping.

Fried eggs are out! Forget Eggs Benedict—except for that rare orange juice and champagne breakfast. No one likes to miss special treats—but we enjoy them more if they are served infrequently and with a constant eye on our health. Keep the fat down and the enjoyment up.

Egg substitutes are formulated foods developed to replace eggs in the diet of those who have high blood cholesterol and are a coronary risk. The formulation is based on doing away with the yolk (which contains the cholesterol) and combining the egg white with a vegetable oil (low in saturates and high in polyunsaturates), a protein, a sugar and a variety of vitamins and minerals to match the composition of the "real" egg. "Egg Beaters," for example, doesn't come in a shell but in a carton. Unlike real egg, it has been pasteurized and homogenized, so that you can only use it in omelettes, in scrambled eggs, or in baked products. It has the same consistency as beaten eggs and has to be frozen to preserve it from spoilage. You'll find it in the freezer section of your supermarket.

Other egg substitutes such as "Eggstra" are formulated much the same except that they are dried. "Eggstra" is made of powdered egg white, powdered whole egg, and powdered milk plus flavor and color. Since it contains small amounts of yolk (part of powdered whole egg), it is not completely free of cholesterol. Also, it is low in fat content as no vegetable oils have been added. To use it for scrambled eggs, baking, or cooking, the powder is re-dissolved.

The choice between these two products will depend on your taste. The difference in nutritional value is small. "Egg Beaters" has more fat, if you need the calories from fat. Otherwise stick to "Eggstra" or similar products.

Fish is good for you. A taste for it should be cultivated in the young so that they pick up the habit. Choose low-fat fish, if possible; steam, poach, or bake—and serve often.

Canned fish is ideal for lunch-time meals, sandwiches, and snacks but there are differences in flavor and nutritional value.

The different names on salmon cans refer to different salmon species. All have about the same nutritional value, but differ in color and quality of the flesh. The most expensive is the deep red salmon, sockeye, which has a slightly higher fat content; the least expensive is the lighter colored chum or keta salmon, with lower fat content. In between these two come the cohoe with a medium red flesh and a lower oil content and the pink salmon which is just that, with fine textured flesh.

The red fleshed salmon is most suitable for serving as is or in salads where appearance is important. The lighter colored and lower priced varieties are suitable for casseroles and other dishes where color isn't important.

The nutritional differences between species are slight. Pink salmon, for example, has more sodium than sockeye salmon, but not enough to count. Salmon is known as a fat fish, but the fat content varies from species to species and also from season to season. The fish with the lower fat content has higher water content so the protein always remains constant.

The different kinds of tuna are actually different species. The most common and the most expensive is the albacore tuna. It has a very white flesh and is usually canned as a solid pack, although it may sometimes be found as a flaked tuna. Skipjack, yellowfin, and bluefin become progressively darker in color and coarser in texture, and are not as readily available in all parts of the country. Bonito and yellowtail are slightly different in texture and flavor. Albacore is the only one which can be called "white meat tuna"; others are "light meat." Tuna may be purchased as solid pack, as chunks and as flakes, or as grated tuna, the scrap ends. The whiter the meat, the more expensive it is. The solid meat is more expensive than the flakes, which are more expensive than the scraps. The solid meat is the first part that is taken out of the fish, and the parts that are left are used up as flakes or scraps. Tuna isn't graded as such, but each packer may produce several brands from the same fish, according to appearance.

Tuna is usually packed with salad oil and a small quantity of salt. The oil may be soya oil, cottonseed oil, or it may be a vegetable broth instead. If it is packed in oil, it is wise to drain it off, especially if you are counting calories. Many types of tuna now have very little oil. If it contains vegetable broth, save and use the liquid if possible because it is rich in nutrients. If you are going to serve the fish right out of the can, or in a dish where color and texture will be noticed, choose the albacore solid pack tuna. For other recipes, the cheapest is just as flavorful and nutritious as the more expensive.

We can effect a major change in the amount of fat we eat by taking the attitude that meat is part of the "act," but not necessarily the star attraction; 3 or 4 ounce (85 to 120 g) servings of meat are large enough. Meat is a very useful, nutritional "go-along" with other foods, such as cereals, legumes, dairy products, fruits, and vegetables, and it "boosts" the nutritional components. Without liver, for example, we would have a much more difficult time balancing budgets and diets. And where would we be without ground beef for hamburgers and casseroles? But you don't need 6 or 8 ounces (as much as 220 g) for one serving; 4 ounces (120 g) will suffice. Always buy lean meat and trim off any fat.

How can we be sure that meat is lean? The trip to the meat counter is a bit of a two-step: It takes you and your butcher to ensure you good quality, low-fat meat of a cut that you recognize and are able to prepare. Learn about both, the characteristics of the various meats and your butcher's expertise.

It is very difficult to judge how much fat is in ground meat just by looking at it, especially if the meat is finely ground, because the juice from the meat tends to cover up the white color of the fat. The fat content regulations are helpful. However, in some places, there are no regulations about how meat should be displayed, so a warm reddish light in the meat display counter may make it look redder than it really is. Sometimes supermarkets line these counters with a nice green frilled paper. Green, as the complementary color of red, also makes the meat look redder than it may really be. If in doubt, ask; don't believe your eyes.

By law, a butcher is not allowed to add fat when he is grinding meat. If you are convinced that your meat is fatter than it should be, save the meat, drippings, and package label. Then write or telephone your local federal or state government inspector and ask him to check it for you. If you must wait several days until he collects it, freeze the contents of the package. He can transport it back to the lab in the frozen state and then analyze it. Butchers who fat-pad the patties are charged and fined.

Luncheon meats such as bologna, sausages, and salamis are sold fresh, cooked, or dried. Whatever the flavor you favor, eat them in moderation if you are concerned about fat and waste.

We do have some indication of the fat content of luncheon meats. In the U.S. the amount of fats in these products is limited to 30 per cent and no more. In Canada, the food and drug regulations specify that the amount of fat should not exceed 40 per cent by weight. This is higher than the upper limit on fat in weiners, which is set at 30 per cent (by weight). In terms of calories, in one slice of bologna, or one hot dog, 70 to 80 per cent of the calories come from *fat*.

A food which has that amount of fat (or more) should be eaten in moderation. Furthermore, it is not a cheap food: consider the amount of water and fillers and compare prices with other cuts of meats.

Balance the convenience of bologna, salami, meat spreads, and hot dogs against their cost in money and health. We remember a letter we received some time ago along with a full can of meat spread. The sender wondered about the hard white stuff on top of the meat.

We wrote back that it was fat, and there was a lot of it. The amount was within the range allowed for meat spreads. Usually, the fat in canned meat spreads is in emulsion. In this can, however—and in fact, in the whole lot—the emulsion had broken and the fat had risen to the top in a hard layer. It must be a common occurrence, but generally the manufacturer stops the cans before they reach the market.

The amount of white stuff on the top was alarming in this case, but it did show that consumer, at least, the amount of fat she ate every time she used the product. The same can be said for bologna or weiners or any of the meat spreads.

What nutrients besides fat are in meat products? Meat products are usually compared with other meat, dairy, or nut products for protein content. Generally, these spreads provide less than half the protein of lean meats. Similarly, Cheddar cheese and peanut butter each contain double or more the protein in meat spreads. At the check-out counter, remember this: At current prices the cost of protein from meat spread is almost two-thirds higher than protein from Cheddar cheese and about four times as much as protein from peanut butter.

How healthful are bologna and weiners? Wasn't there some question about bacteria in weiners a while back? Weiners came under scrutiny by the U.S. Consumers' Union, which strongly recommended cooking the meat for at least five minutes in boiling water and 20 minutes under the broiler to kill the bacteria.

As for bologna, processors vacuum-pack it in hermetically sealed containers and the government requires the label to state "keep refrigerated," and "perishable." The vacuum-packaging process does not include heating after packaging. Thus, if food-poisoning bacteria that can grow and multiply without air are present in the meat at the time of packaging, toxins (poisons) can be produced if this product is held at room temperature.

If the vacuum-packaged meat is kept refrigerated, toxins will not form. It is possible to hold some vacuum-packaged foods, such as bologna, for many days at room temperature without apparent spoilage, but "apparent" is the key word. The product will not have any off-odor, nor will it appear spoiled. Therefore, we will not know, until a queasy stomach begins, whether the product contained any toxins.

The guarantee of safety rests with the handling and storage methods used by the food processor, the retailer, and us. Unfortunately, the chain may be weak at some point. During transport from processor to retailer, refrigerated storage may be less than optimum. Some retailers may abuse meat products packaged in air-impermeable plastic pouches by displaying them at store temperatures rather than keeping them refrigerated.

We have to be careful not to leave purchases in the back of a car on a warm day for any length of time, and to place vacuum-packaged meats promptly in the refrigerator. Sandwiches prepared from these re-frigerated meats may be carried in a lunch box and eaten a few hours later without any hazard.

Buy your bologna in a store that has a big turnover and use it quickly. Don't buy more than you will use before your next shopping trip, and never buy a package that is bloated, has milky slime inside the package, or has any leaks in the plastic.

Then there are meatless sausages, links, and patties. These are made from textured soy protein alone or in combination with other proteins, such as wheat gluten and egg albumen.

One example of these products is the Morningstar Farms breakfast links, patties, and slices. They are packaged like breakfast sausages and ham slices and are kept frozen.

Such products usually contain polyunsaturated vegetable oil instead of saturated meat fat, no cholesterol, and a lower fat content than meat. They also have a favorable P/S ratio and quantity and quality of protein comparable to meat.

What about margarines and oils? The blending of oil with butter as described in Chapter 4 gives a suitable substitute for butter and margarine. There are going to be occasions, however, when blended butter is not available and you'll need to buy margarine. Here's how.

All labels of margarines and oils are required, by regulations, to carry a declaration of the type of oil they contain; e.g., vegetable oil or marine (fish) oil.

Manufacturers are required to say whether or not the oil is hydrogenated or just partially so. Often the label states the amounts of saturated and polyunsaturated fats. In this case, always ensure that you have at least as much polyunsaturated fat as you do saturated fat. The least amount of hydrogenation is the most desirable.

Hard margarines have very little to commend them except price. They are made of combinations of marine and/or vegetable oils and have been hydrogenated to a high saturation level.

Soft margarine has more polyunsaturates than saturates and is labelled accordingly. That is fairly simple to understand. But there is also whipped margarine or butter, which contains "less" fat. For these, air is whipped into the spread to give it more volume and less fat per spoonful. Be sure to examine the label—only if the polyunsaturates are higher than the saturates will the margarine be helpful in controlling the risk of high blood cholesterol.

To spray or not to stick. As we said in Chapter 4, we recommend browning stewing meat in hard fat, chilling it to allow the fat to congeal and removing the surface excess before reheating to serve. We also recommend small amounts of oil for quick pan-broiling. But what of the no–stick sprays?

No-stick aerosol sprays which you apply to cooking utensils to prevent food from sticking contain only two ingredients: lecithin and a propellant, usually a freon gas. Different manufacturers use a different formula for each ingredient. Taste and odor vary, depending on the form of lecithin and gas used.

Pure lecithin is harmless, but at room temperature it is quite heavy and viscous. It needs a lot of propellant to send it out of the can, and consequently the no-stick sprays usually contain only 10 per cent lecithin with 90 per cent propellant. The gas is odorless and apparently dissipates when it leaves the can.

Environmentalists are concerned about the increased use of propellants and question the saturation point of the earth's atmosphere in relationship to these gases. Health professionals question the safety of daily use to the health of the individual.

So while the occasional use of such a spray would not harm us, constant and increased use poses a threat. We cannot recommend it.

Teflon pans, on the other hand, offer an excellent no-stick, no-fat method of cooking without the disadvantages of the sprays. We recomend these highly.

As American as apple pie—as Canadian as butter tarts. In our scheme of dining, there is a place for desserts of fruits and nuts, cheese and crackers—even an occasional slice of angel cake with a sauce of hot cherries in Kirsch. We choose pies or cakes only occasionally. But for the odd time (at Hallowe'en when we've done everything with the pumpkin—pickled it, "puddinged" it, and eaten the seeds) when we serve a hot pie, making the pie crust takes particular care. Here shortening is necessary for good results.

The vegetable shortenings on the market today are made by hydrogenating an oil. As with margarine, this means that hydrogen atoms are added to the fatty acid molecules to solidify the oil and make it hard at room temperature.

There is evidence to suggest that the formation of the trans-form of fatty acid occurs during hydrogenation. This form of fatty acids has been shown to contribute to high blood cholesterol levels. So until we can be convinced that this danger is adequately regulated we will look to other unprocessed fats for pastry making.

Oil (or if hard shortening is required, lard) are our choices for baked goods.

The blended butter recipe given in Chapter 4 is excellent for baking but could be expensive if you bake a lot. A combination of lard and oil is cheaper. It has the advantage of having an acceptable P/S ratio and, not to be discounted, the quality to make a very fine pie!

PERFECT PASTRY

2-crust pie or 2 single-crust pies, for 8" (20 cm) pie pans
2 cups (500 mL) cake and pastry flour (sift and measure)
⅓ cup (75 mL) lard
¼ cup (50 mL) (safflower, sunflower or corn)
3 tbsp. (50 mL) water
¼ tsp. (1 mL) salt (optional)

Measure sifted flour into a bowl. Cut lard into flour with pastry blender until it is the size of small peas. Mix oil, water and salt. Add to the flour mixture. Toss with a fork until it forms a ball. Roll pastry as you would for your favorite recipes. Fill and bake as susual.

Convenience products are the custom today, regardless of whether you work at or away from home. We have come to rely on canned soup, ketchup, processed cheese slices, and other convenience foods as staples in our refrigerators. Convenience foods account for a large portion of our food dollar. They are here to stay and will proliferate in the years to come.

Many ordinary foods such as eggs, meat, fish, poultry, vegetables, fruits, and cereals are convenient. They can be served simply and are cheaper, more wholesome and easier than any "convenience" foods on the market. A taste for simple food can be your greatest convenience.

Look critically at any convenience foods you do buy and compare the saving in time and effort with the cost in food value and money. The problem is that we seldom have all the facts. We would dearly love to be able to place every item which purports to being convenient into a neat nutritional category with a rating for each product, but they change too often. But we can make some general recommendations if you are in need of "convenience" and speed of preparation and wish to have every bit of nourishment available.

There is considerable information about the effect of processing on the vitamin and mineral content of foods, and we know that there is a loss of vitamins and minerals at each step of processing. So:

Rule #1. Buy convenience foods that have had a minimum amount of handling. Frozen or canned peas which you cook quickly in a minimum of water are going to retain more nutrients than the frozen peas in a TV dinner which have been blanched, cooked, frozen and slowly reheated in the oven. Canned chicken is going to be much more nourishing in a sauce you make yourself than in a fat-laden chicken pot pie which has been heated, drenched in sauce, frozen and reheated. A macaroni to which you add your own cheese will be a more delicious form of nourishment than the one to which you add a powdered mix.

Rule #2. Never consider convenience "dinners" or "meals" to be complete. When we compared the nutritional adequacy of some commercial TV dinners with what nutrients we expect to get from a meal, we found that they were low in calories, calcium, and riboflavin. These "dinners" or "meals" may be used occasionally through the week (once or twice) but *always* served with milk and a green salad, and for a teenager, add several slices of whole grain bread and butter to give him the energy he needs.

Rule #3. Avoid foods with long lists of ingredients. A food is a food is a food. The longer the list, the more ingredients in a processed food, the greater likelihood that you will have nutrient dilution to the point where you are paying more of your hard-earned dollars for fewer calories and little nourishment.

Rule #4. Convenience foods cost more, so make sure that you buy those which are "best buys." U.S. Department of agriculture figures indicate that of 16 frozen convenience main courses, 10 were more expensive than their home-prepared counterparts. A survey by the Consumers' Association of Canada on one convenience food, "frozen fish and chips," found that the maid-service in the package (the difference between the cost of ingredients and the item) accounted for more than two-thirds of its cost. When buying a product like this (if you do it at all!) make certain that there is more fish than chips and more fish than batter. If you're dissatisfied, return it!

A microwave oven is a great convenience. In the past, safety was a concern, but today a microwave oven is as safe to use in your kitchen as a blender. The government regulations and the fail-safe mechanisms on the ovens themselves ensure that there is no radiation leakage. The problem seems to come when the door seam seal weakens, either through careless use or food buildup. The new ovens are constructed so that at the slightest leak, the unit goes off. Old ovens in use in public places are now (or should be) inspected often for such leakage.

The microwave oven can free a family from the necessity of using prepared, processed foods and can allow a return to fresh foods. Oatmeal porridge cooks in seconds in your own bowl; vegetables and meats cook right on the plate.

If you're shopping for an oven, look at the instruction booklet and make certain that it gives times and information for all quantities of foods. Any microwave recipe book should tell you times for all foods as well as for varying amounts of each.

The microwave oven frees you from the weekend casserole cook-and-freeze pattern. Just a few years back, a working person who wanted good meals through the week had to prepare, cook, freeze all weekend for the week to come or, alternatively, rely on processed foods. A microwave oven allows you to buy fresh foods such as meat, potatoes, vegetables, and fruits in season, and cook and serve them in half an hour. A roast of beef, a dressed fish, hamburgers, rice, and vegetables can all be prepared in less than an hour, with a minimum of nutrient loss!

The most convenient appliance of all is another person. As more homes have several working members, it becomes more important that everyone has a say and a share in the food shopping and preparation.

It's in everyone's best interest to eat well and it should be everyone's responsibility. In our homes all members participate in planning the menus, shopping, and preparation.

It requires a change of attitude for some people. Change is ongoing, however, and for the sake of good health and family co-operation, it becomes essential. Liberate the men and the boys so they'll learn and enjoy a creative art! After a busy day at the office, many hands can make light (and rewarding) work.

REMEMBER

Master the supermarket game! Use NutriScore.

Let the produce counter be your guide to meal planning.

Fresh is best but canned and frozen without sugar are excellent substitutes when fresh fruits and vegetables look like they'll break the budget.

Switch to oil. Oil is best for eating, baking, dressing salads and sandwiches.

Of the 150 cereals on the market shelf, less than half a dozen provide the natural nourishment a cereal should. Cooked, unrefined cereals are cheapest and best for you. Uncooked, unrefined whole-grain cereals are good, too. Don't waste money on sugared, highly processed breakfast "cereals".

Use skim milk—powdered is especially convenient. Choose low-fat cheeses and substitute yogurt for sour cream.

Eggs are too good to miss. Youngsters need them often, oldsters need them too. Three to four eggs a week for adults and seven to ten eggs each week for the under-20s.

Consider fish, poultry, lentils, beans, and nuts as dollars and cents-ible replacements for beef, pork, and lamb. Use them often.

Don't pay protein prices for fat. Buy lean meat and use only three to four ounces (120 g) for one serving.

There are four rules of convenience food buying: Avoid over priced convenience. Avoid over-processed convenience. Avoid "whole dinners" unless you plan to balance your meals yourself. Avoid convenience when it comes in packages with long ingredient lists.

Be flexible. Choose nutritious foods that you can prepare comfortably, with a minimum of fuss and fat, and a maximum of nutrition and enjoyment.

Chapter 17

Eating Out Can Be Nourishing

Not very long ago eating out meant a treat on a special occasion. A celebration for whatever reason was usually marked by dinner "on the town."

Today, it is almost an everyday occurrence. More of us dine out than ever before.

Who is responsible for your nutrition when eating out? No one but yourself. You are on your own. Formerly the wife and mother controlled what went into family lunch boxes, but now she can only suggest healthful food for the family to buy and hope it's available. Schools provide space but usually lease out the cafeteria and vending machine concessions and won't interfere with them. Concessionaires stock what they can be sure of selling. Lunch truck and restaurant owners do the same. The government lays down regulations prohibiting the sale of unclean or noxious foods but says nothing about meals that couldn't possibly add up to good health. And the food manufacturers keep bringing out newer, more refined, less nourishing products every day. Simple, unrefined, wholesome foods are becoming hard to find in eating-out places. No one is watching to see that we get our money's worth of nourishment.

Here is where NutriScore can really help. Use it to plan your day's menu. Once you know what areas need strengthening, you can plan the foods you want to choose (or leave out) when the menu is placed before you. Careful before-hand planning avoids those last-minute mistakes.

Children and teenagers need the most help in eating nutritiously away from home. Even when they have been accustomed to good food and have come to enjoy the sensible meals served at the family table, they tend to lose their judgment among peers. Confronted with a lot of persuasively advertised junk, they lack the maturity to see it as a potential health hazard. Many a well-fed child has thrown out the nourishing lunch from home to spend his allowance on forbidden fruit (i.e., pop and chips) from the vending machine.

Use NutriScore at breakfast to point out the good choices the youngsters need that day.

Schools, looking for fast service and economy, often shift from nutritionally balanced cafeteria meals to vending machines or nothing at all.

It needn't be so. A concerned mother in Bloomington, Indiana, rallied other parents and put a stop to vending machines selling junk food in their school system. After two years of patient labor and discouragement, they achieved total victory when the school board voted a complete ban on junk food in schools.

What made the ban significant was that Monroe County was in financial straits and needed the money. It was the worst possible time to cut out precious vending machine revenues. Yet, the school board went ahead with the ban and refused to pad the budget by selling junk foods. The school board president stated, "We will not provide a facility for private enterprise to come in and sell foods which are not nutritionally valuable and make a profit on our school children." He observed that children had been spending their lunch money on soda-pop and candy, and so going without a nutritious meal. And Bloomington was just the beginning. Now many school boards have acted to outlaw sugar-loaded foods and to require vendors to include some nutritious foods in school vending machines.

Obviously, angry parents can do a great deal, but not without the help of the school principal. Hooray for the head of a New Haven, Connecticut, school who sent a letter home at the beginning of the school year advising parents that junk foods such as potato chips, candy, soda-pop would not be sold nor tolerated in school lunches.

The board of education of one of our local boroughs could do with a few of that principal's principles. A friend of ours discovered that her three children were having a mid-morning doughnut break. She telephoned their principal, "Why a doughnut break, for goodness sake?" "Well," he replied, "we have found that youngsters have a slump mid-morning and need some food energy." "Yes," she agreed, "but why doughnuts?" "Well, for instant energy," was the reply. "Bosh! milk breaks, yes. When I was a child during the war, we had milk at recesses; even back then everyone recognized the need for mid-morning snacks. But doughnuts are full of fat and sugar and low in food value. What are you teaching these children of mine? Is my twelve-year-old going to look for a doughnut every time she feels low?"

There are no nutritional standards for the foods sold in restaurants or by the catering industry. As long as it's sanitary and isn't falsely advertised, the government agencies appointed to protect us appear to be happy.

The food service and catering industry rely on polls and market research in deciding what to sell. They take no part in helping the public get adequate nourishment. They want to make money by filling demands and perpetuating these demands. This summation is often that the public's main requirement of the food industry is reasonable price. One can hardly blame businessmen for filling this demand. One can, however, ask whether the public is not confidently assuming that cheap food will also be nourishing, and if the food industry is not breaking faith with its customers at this point. Who knows better than the caterers themselves that the meals they prepare lack nutritional value and present dangers to health?

The restaurant and food service industry concentrates a good deal of effort on studying our spending habits and characterizing the high profit profile on each menu item. This is sound marketing. However, we cannot expect much improvement in the nutritional quality of restaurant foods if this factor assumes top priority.

These days the number of "health food" restaurants and cafeterias is on the increase. This must reflect consumer demand, for when it comes to marketing food, business is sensitive to our moods. It is possible that our insistence on quality, both in food and service, may gradually affect our eating places. Chefs and food managers will soon learn that fast food can be prepared without sacrificing the nutrition the consumer wants.

Which are the best food choices from a vending machine? If the machine offers you the typical selection of chocolate bars, cookies, and chips, cookies are probably the best alternative. Chips are high in fat and salt. Chocolate bars are often about the same in calories as cookies, but have more sugar.

When it comes to beverages, most vending machines offer a choice of hot ones such as coffee, tea, or maybe hot chocolate; or a choice of cold soft drinks. All these beverages come plain or with sugar and/or non-dairy whitener or cream. The soft drinks are basically carbonated, colored, and flavored sugar solutions. An easy way out of paying for empty calories is to reach for the nearest fountain or tap where water is dispensed free of charge and free of calories.

Certainly, if the machine offers milk, muffins, and fresh fruit your choice is very much simpler. Any or all of these would be wise, and a combination would be even better.

Restaurant cooking methods are chosen for their speed and adaptation to streamline production. There is widespread use of frying as the choice method for cooking in restaurants. It is fast. Food takes less time to fry than to boil or bake. The oil sustains higher temperatures than boiling water or an oven. Frying means that there can be continuous cooking. Oil doesn't evaporate if maintained at the right temperature and frying lends itself to the addition of flavors and seasonings which can be blended to cover the bland taste of some food.

Fried foods add to our fat consumption. Further, heating oil to a very high temperature in deep-frying results in chemical changes and the production of substances that may interfere with digestion and absorption of foods.

Many studies in recent years have shown that the most popular item on a restaurant menu is french fried potatoes. It is difficult to find a restaurant or cafeteria line that does not serve french fries. In fact, it is often difficult to order a sandwich without getting french fries and being charged for them. Their popularity becomes self-perpetuating. (We mentioned the nutritional drawbacks of french fries in Chapters 8 and 15.)

French frying is not restricted to potatoes. Notice the popularity of french fried onion rings, fried chicken, and fried fish. The proliferation of fried food in restaurants has reached such a point that many restaurants sell digestive aids, in anticipation of distress. Bromo Seltzer sits right by the cash register!

Don't count on the oil used in frying for much besides fat. The oil industry is not unaware of the criticism of the wide use of frying. Much of the advertising for cooking oils emphasizes the relatively small amount absorbed by the food. The oil people and the manu-facturers of deep-frying equipment have worked out the precise conditions for frying foods to reduce the uptake of oil. These conditions specify the exact temperature for heating and maintaining oil, the length of time it may be used, and when to discard it. Oil is processed and purified to enhance its cooking stability under severe heat treatment. This may require the manufacturers to fractionate it, which often removes essential nutrients (such as vitamin E). Such purification practices can have serious nutritional consequences. If a person is determined to live on fried foods, it would be nice to see him get all the vitamins possible.

Fresh fruits and vegetables are too expensive to be profitable for restaurants to serve and, because they spoil easily, wastage is high. As a result, potatoes are nearly always instant, and apples show up only in apple pies. Even coleslaw usually sits around losing nourishment, sometimes longer than the succotash.

Restaurants favor the use of convenience foods much more than housewives do. Many convenience foods are produced and packed for institution use long before they are introduced on the retail market. Those who eat out frequently can expect to be served orange-flavored drinks under the banner of orange juice, instant in place of mashed potatoes, pre-cooked oatmeal instead of regular porridge, and non-dairy coffee whitener rather than milk or cream in coffee or tea.

Restaurant meals can be good for you, if you have the detemination and persistence to eat only at those places that offer the nutritional choices you want.

Many restaurants rely on pre-packaged entrées, prepared elsewhere and re-heated in microwave ovens when the customer places the order at the table. We wouldn't be surprised if many more restaurants eventually will eliminate the chef and kitchen altogether and replace them with banks of computerized billing centers and microwave ovens, backed by freezers and fast delivery services.

We first suspected that our chic neighborhood restaurant was operating an ersatz eatery when the ham-asparagus quiche arrived burning hot. It was much hotter than any quiche baked in an oven at home. We quickly presumed pre-packaging. Upon inspection, we were proved right. Green plants in the dining room, charm, decor, and Vivaldi coming from the loud speakers—but no chef in the kitchen.

What's wrong with this? Nothing, beyond our values and taste buds, goes the argument. But, since most dishes are prepared in heavy sauces so they can be frozen and reheated, the long cooking will probably destroy the nutrients, and the sauces will be high in calories. If you rely upon restaurant meals for half or one-third of your daily calories, you would probably be putting on pounds while losing nutrition.

Furthermore, to whom do we complain when there is no chef to stand behind the quality and presentation of the food?

To get what you want from a restaurant, you must ask. You can always get milk instead of cream for your coffee or tea or cereal and thereby receive not only a more nourishing product but also a safer one: you'll get less fat, and bypass the non-dairy coffee whiteners made with coconut oil and cream that has been out of the refrigerator all day.

Don't hesitate to ask for substitutes when ordering complete dinners—a boiled or baked potato instead of french fries or a tossed salad in place of a vegetable you don't like.

Remember to order no gravy on meat and potatoes, have the salad dressing brought to the table (so that you can control the amount to be added), order your dessert without whipped cream, (or skip dessert altogether). You can control the calories and fat and thus your enjoyment of the meal.

Complete dinners are often too generous. Most menus offer choices of complete dinners, all of them with hors d'oeuvres, appetizers, main course, and dessert. The price is high and there is more food than you can or should eat. Many times we have asked the maitre d' (often to his controlled horror) for soup, salad, and a cheese tray. The cost is reasonable and still leaves us feeling satisfied, but not overly full.

The cafeteria offers self-service, but often foods are arranged in such a way as to influence your choice adversely. Have you noticed how all cafeteria lines start with desserts? While your hunger for food is the greatest, you are faced with a decision on dessert first. Unless you are familiar with the particular cafeteria and have decided in advance what you want and where to find it, it is difficult to choose wisely in a busy cafeteria line. Impulse buying becomes the rule. We advise you not to allow this to happen. Case the joint first, and choose what you want before you pick up your tray. After all, it's your stomach and it should be treated carefully.

There are usually excellent choices in cafeterias. Follow the same principles which guide you in planning nourishing meals at home and you'll be fine. There is usually a decent choice of meat sandwiches, various salads, fresh fruit, and cottage cheese. Most people's difficulties arise when they reach for the lemon meringue pie instead of yogurt. However, if you eat regularly in cafeterias the temptation to choose junk foods decreases with familiarity. The yogurt often tastes better than the phony lemon, phony meringue, pasty-tasting pie.

One young mother we know found she was over-spending both calories and money when she ate lunch in the department store cafeteria on her weekly outing. She solved both problems by choosing a bowl of vegetable soup (the cafeteria's specialty), a small carrot salad (which her family didn't particularly enjoy, so she seldom made it at home) a whole wheat roll, a square of cheese and a glass of skim milk. She often ate this lunch before twelve, shopped while the noon-hour crowd was in the cafeteria, and went back herself around three to have a fruit salad or fresh fruit or ice cream and a cup of coffee before she returned to face the fray at home.

We won't say you'll eat as well in a cafeteria as at home, but we think you will have a chance of good nutrition there, if you combine the elements of the meal properly.

Fast food meals account for more than one-quarter of all meals eaten away from home. Dr. Paul LaChance of Rutgers University in New Brunswick, New Jersey, published data on the nutritive value of the meals available from McDonalds, Kentucky Fried Chicken, Dairy Queen, and Burger King. He found that the best available nutritional combination was a large or super-size burger with or without cheese. But even a burger with chips and a soft drink was low in calcium, vitamin A and vitamin C. The same burger with chips and milk instead of a soft drink would be improved in calcium, protein, riboflavin, and niacin. Vitamins A and C would still be inadequate.

A meal of Kentucky Fried Chicken, coleslaw and a roll could not be considered adequate as it is deficient in calcium, iron, vitamin A, thiamin, riboflavin, and vitamin C.

The picture, while gloomy, isn't hopeless. As long as you're aware that you need sources of vitamin A and vitamin C and trace minerals and vitamins such as folic acid, you can make up for them in other meals.

But, don't neglect them! Vitamin C is essential in our bodies' protection mechanisms, vitamin A keeps the bloom on our epithelial, cells, and both ward off aggressive viral and bacterial intruders.

Our suggestion "if you deserve that break today" would be to choose the large burger (without the chips, if you can't afford the calories) and say "no" to the soft drink and take milk instead. Make sure you have a good large green salad at lunch and a large orange or a glass of orange juice at breakfast. Check NutriScore, too, for other foods that can balance your day for you.

Movie theaters and roadside stands also sell foods. Recently, on a children's matinee day at the local theater we were intrigued watching the youngsters choose their snacks. Most took candy or popcorn and pop (all nutritionally empty) but some chose pre-cooked, pre-wrapped and warmed weiners in buns. As the throng thinned, I asked the girl how she cooked them. She explained that she left them on the heated rollers for about 5 to 10 minutes until they had split (and my eyes were sound enough to see that they hadn't even done that!), and then she removed them to the roll, to the foil envelope and thence to the warming oven.

Ouch! Even if they have been cooked for long enough (20 minutes, according to laboratory tests) to kill bacteria, the temperature in the holding ovens is not high enough to retard the growth of food poisoning bacteria. It may not be more than a tiny stomach ache, but why spoil a movie because of intestinal malaise? Better to opt for peanuts or seeds, and leave the hot dogs on the rollers.

Barbecue-cooked chickens that you buy for re-heating should go from the rotisserie straight home to the oven (if served hot) or the refrigerator (if served cold). In either case, always choose a chicken that has just been freshly barbecued, not one that has been sitting for hours in a warming oven.

Nothing loves a chicken as much as bacteria, especially if the chicken is at room temperature or slightly warmer. Your refrigerator will not object to having a hot chicken made suddenly cold. It's designed to do just that, so use it!

What choice do you have at parties? The most obvious way to get out of eating too much at friends' homes is to talk your way out of it. We have a friend who, for religious and health reasons, cannot eat certain foods. Because she's a naturally outgoing and friendly person, she never refuses a dinner invitation. However, once confronted with foods she must avoid she simply carries on talking and cutting food and moving it about from place to place on her plate ever so skillfully and no one notices that she is not eating much. She follows up her performance by helping clear the table and clean up.

We certainly don't advocate such drastic measures. However, her example could serve to put the delights of "eating out" in perspective. Let's remember that it's the company and conversation which makes dining with friends special. Good food, well prepared, enhances the pleasure of a convivial gathering. The dinner itself should be considered as the garnish rather than the main course.

If you have a specific allergy, advise the hostess ahead of time. A friend of ours who has an allergic reaction to shellfish makes it a practice to tell the hostess well in advance. It saves embarrassment later and really does help the hostess plan her menu.

What should you serve? Hostessing is an art of a special sort. How to attend to the food and drink while still having time to partake of enjoyable conversation has always been a challenge. But modern homemakers have mastered it, mostly with pre-preparation, careful planning and casseroles. Good nutrition can be included in the planning as well. For dinner parties, we plan only one drink beforehand and make that a light wine if possible. The hors d'oeuvre is a green salad often served with grapefruit or orange sections and some homemade rye or seasoned melba toast. The main course needn't be heavy. Served with two or three brightly colored vegetables freshly cooked and seasoned, it can be a delight to both the palate and the eye. What about chicken breasts lighly browned and served with a sprinkle of lemon or pineapple juice? In our opinion and that of the greatest chefs anywhere, vegetable cookery is a grand art. So, we like to concentrate on last-minute cooking of vegetables. Thin strips of carrots that have been prepared or cooked until tender are tossed with tiny bits of mint and chopped parsley. They look and taste delicious, especially when served with a green vegetable.

After all, anyone can cook a steak, but only the most careful and conscientious hostess will trouble to think about the color and texture of those heavenly vegetables. Dessert comes in two courses in our houses, the first course is a light homemade sherbet or meringue with fruit or lemon sauce, and the second course is a bowl of fresh fruit, a plate of cheese, and a bowl of walnuts.

The art of hostessing must take into consideration the state of the nation's avoirdupois. With more than half of us overweight, a hostess should remember to reduce the sauces and rich desserts, the heavily buttered breads and creamy pies that would contribute to a person's girth in favor of more delicate, light foods. Guests with allergies or religious constraints have no room for indecision, but most of the rest of us are ambivalent. The hostess must bear the responsibility for her choice of foods and therefore for her guests' enjoyment. If we assume that good health is one factor in enjoyment then we can arrange to serve dinners that are modest, tasteful, and nourishing.

We plan parties, such as the late night buffet, or supper after a show or a children's birthday, with the same regard for health. Do all the guests really want hunks of bread to dip in the cheese fondue or should there be celery sticks and other vegetables for dipping, too? Cake and coffee is a nice way to round out an evening. Most of us by now have recognized that coffee affects us in one way or another, and many hostesses do provide the decaffeinated coffee for guests who don't like a late night brew. In the same way, a hostess will not be insulted if you ask for a small piece of cake and enjoy it very much.

What's a birthday party without a cake and candles? Nobody says it has to be large, though, or that everybody has to eat some. In our experience children often eat less at parties, although anyone who counts on anything going the way she expects at a birthday party hasn't been a mother very long. Anyway, you don't need a lot of rich food to celebrate. At one time chicken à la king was considered appropriate party fare, but the effect is hardly worthwhile—the kids are usually too excited to eat. Nowadays the favored birthday foods are sandwiches, hot dogs, and hamburgers. A thoughtful mother lightens the heavy taste with carrot sticks, celery, cherry tomatoes and so on. And a plate of devilled eggs goes surprisingly fast. (Leave the paprika off half of them though; there are some finicky kids around.) Another hit-maker is pineapple wedges on toothpicks served in the pineapple shell. Children think of such dishes as something served at adult parties, so they're a real treat.

Incidentally, when your children go to more parties on their own, they'll need a little warning about eating small helpings and suggestions about which choice is best.

And then there's Christmas and Easter and Thanksgiving. These are all times for celebration with food, course upon course upon course of food. Traditionally, we're expected to be gluttonous on these days. But, it's time now that we came to our senses. These occasions were never meant to be the time to force heavy rich food on family members. There are too many underfed around our world and too many overfed around our tables. Any religious holiday or family gathering is exciting and pleasant by itself. A modest, attractive meal, in keeping with the tradition of the occasion, would make it even more meaningful.

"What would you like to drink?" This is the first question from a hospitable host. It surely is an indication of the part that alcohol plays in our society that the general term "drink" is understood to mean alcohol.

For many people, the end of a working day is celebrated with a drink. For some, a drink or two at noon before lunch is part of the business day routine. Others rely on a drink to put them sleep for the night or to put them at ease for a social or business function.

In moderation, alcohol exerts positive effects on many people. It relaxes nerves and muscles. Social gatherings are enjoyable with everyone in a relaxed state. But the key to enjoyment is not drinking any more than your body can handle. Like any good thing, alcohol is harmful in excess.

So, know your own capacity. Excessive drinking is a state that may vary from one individual to another and can be affected by body size. This is not surprising since a large person has a greater blood volume and a larger liver and may be able to handle more alcohol than a small person. Each person should determine the number of drinks at any one time and per day beyond which he experiences changes in mood or stomach queasiness or head lightness. For most people, it takes one or two drinks to feel a change in mood. For some, it is often less than one drink.

Use a jigger. A friend of ours has always been generous in handing down drinks to his guests. By the time the first course is served a number of guests are no longer in a condition to appreciate it. On one occasion, a guest who knew that the dessert had been one of his favorites admitted later that he had no recollection of eating it. That guest presented the host with a thank-you gift. It was a clearly marked shot glass. You certainly don't need to wait for such hints. A good drink is a carefully measured drink.

A very simple technique to avoid over-drinking at a party is to shift to the mix after the first drink. If your first drink was whiskey and soda, you can make your second, third, and fourth just soda water. You will stay more sociable longer and you will enjoy yourself during and after the party.

Don't drink on an empty stomach. In the presence of fats and proteins in the stomach, alcohol absorption is slowed down so that it trickles into the blood stream and into the liver in small amounts. Nuts and crackers and cheese are good companions to a drink, but don't go for the salted variety in case they make you thirsty and send you back for a refill too soon.

Make the drinks last, again so that the liver has time to do its work. A low calorie long drink is vermouth and soda with a twist of lime. Or, if you like it a bit tangier, try vermouth and tonic.

Watch your alcohol intake if you have a physical illness or are on medication. Always ask a physician if you can drink under these circumstances. Since alcohol tends to dissolve blood clots, it irritates ulcer sites and can bring about bouts of bleeding, so ulcer sufferers are usually warned off alcohol. Other effects are not so noticeable as bleeding, but be prepared for odd reactions when alcohol is introduced to metabolic disturbances or to the chemicals in pills.

Remember that not all drinks agree with everybody. There are a number of chemicals formed or added in the fermentation and bottling of various alcoholic beverages. And the drinks themselves are made from various source materials. We know a young boy who, whenever he tussles on the lawn with his pals and grazes the juniper bush, breaks out in a rash. It's quite possible that he will someday develop the same rash from the gin made from juniper. A friend of ours consistently gets a migraine headache after wine and cheese parties. Another friend can drink (in small amounts, mind you) anything except the red wine put out by one company; it makes her sick every time. When you "name your poison," name what suits you and your purposes best.

The key to happy drinking is good nutrition and moderation with alcohol. Develop your strategy before you go to the next cocktail party; stay close to the food, shift to mixes after the first drink. Above all, enjoy yourself and stay in touch with the real world.

REMEMBER

There are no nutritional standards for the foods that are sold in restaurants or by catering companies. It falls to you to control the quality of the nourishment in your foods. Choose healthfully; maintain a good NutriScore rating.

Schools have a responsibility to offer good food in the cafeteria and proper nutrition education in the classroom. If your school falls short in either area, be concerned; get involved in changing things.

Restaurant foods are often fried, over-processed, and lacking in optimum nutritional value. Refuse these and favor non-fatty, natural foods. Restaurateurs will soon get the message.

Kentucky Fried Chicken and Big Macs are O.K. occasionally—but they need balancing. Use NutriScore areas B to F foods in addition.

Entertaining with an eye to good nutrition is IN—gluttony is OUT.

Plan for eating and drinking. It's your good health you're thinking about.

Chapter 18

Nutrition in the Drugstore

Now that you've mastered your diet with NutriScore, you may want to learn more about the pharmaceutical products you use and whether or not they affect the way foods are used in the body. Some preparations in the drugstore contribute to our nourishment and many affect how we use the nutrients in our foods. Vitamin and mineral supplements give us nutrients. Laxatives and diuretics can wash out a lot of nutrients from our bodies.

Everyone knows that drugs affect the body, but not everyone considers the way the state of the body can affect the way it uses these medications. To get the most benefit from any medication it is essential to use it in the right quantity for the body size; to know whether to take it with food as you do with aspirin or without food as you do with some antibiotics; and to know if alcohol interferes with the medication, as it does with some tranquilizers.

Physicians are trained to take all these factors into account when prescribing drugs. They usually are aware of the nutritional side effects of long-term drug therapy and will advise you how to cope with them. But they may not bother to tell you much about occasional drugs, so don't be afraid to ask when and what you should drink and eat.

At the non-prescription drug counter you're on your own. Most painkillers, cold relievers, antacids, laxatives, and vitamin and mineral supplements are not considered dangerous enough to warrant medical guidance; but you'll get plenty of guidance from the advertiser. In choosing and using preparatory drugs don't believe everything you hear. And, while convincing words may flow out of the mouth of an attractive model in an advertisement, just make sure you know what is going into yours.

Are you, or is anyone you know, on the Pill? If so you may need to increase your intake of folic acid and other B vitamins. One recent study described two patients on oral contraceptives who developed megaloblastic anemia affecting the levels of hemoglobin in the blood, as well as the levels of folic acid and vitamin B_{12}. Several other studies show that the mental depression sometimes associated with oral contraceptives is eased by the intake of vitamin B_6. It is possible that further nutritional side effects of the Pill will be discovered as time goes on. This does not mean oral contraceptives are nutritionally harmful, only that you should be aware of undesirable effects and counteract them. Women on the Pill should make sure they have an adequate supply of the B vitamins by eating liver, meat, milk, and whole-grain cereals more often. They should seek a physician's advice if they think they need a vitamin supplement.

Do you use diuretics? These are popularly called "water pills," their purpose being to increase the urine output. If you receive them regularly, your doctor should prescribe a potassium supplement to make up for the potassium loss. Sometimes doctors do not prescribe any supplement or advise a change in diet when the diuretic therapy is for occasional use, such as to relieve menstrual tension caused by excessive fluid in the tissues. On the other hand, if you're feeling weak, lackadaisical, and inefficient it may strike you as well worth the trouble to eat extra bananas or tomatoes or take a few potassium pills for the short time you use the diuretic in order to retain your normal bounce. Do not diagnose yourself, but if pills for water retention deplete your energy tell the doctor who prescribed them and ask whether additional potassium would help.

Cholesterol-lowering agents are new drugs and not everybody knows that when they bind bile acids and bile salts they also cause a loss of fat-soluble vitamins. It's worthwhile to ask your physician whether you need extra vitamins while you are taking these drugs.

Vitamin and mineral supplements are not normally necessary. If you eat a balanced diet (and with the aid of the rating system in Chapter 2 you can make sure that your diet *is* balanced) then you have no need for further vitamins and minerals. However, in case of illness or medication causing nutritional imbalances, a supplement may be needed. In such cases, your physician is the person to decide what you lack and prescribe the specific vitamins and minerals that you need. If you are prevented by allergies, strong dislikes, or moral convictions from eating a balanced diet, you may have to resort to a vitamin and/or mineral supplement. The choice of supplement should be discussed with your doctor with the help of a dietitian or nutritionist. The amounts of each of the vitamins and/or minerals in the supplement need not exceed the levels given in Chapter 7. It is crucial that you have only the vitamins and/or minerals that you are missing in your diet and only in the amounts you need—not more and not less. Taking too much of certain vitamins and minerals is sometimes as dangerous as taking too little. If the body is designed to handle a certain level of a vitamin or mineral, presenting it with more than it can handle means that some tissue or part of the body is going to be poisoned with the excess.

Painkillers usually contain acetylsalicylic acid, which we know as aspirin or a.s.a. This drug has been observed over many years to cause occasional bleeding in the stomach wall, particularly when taken shortly before or after the consumption of alcohol.

It is preferable to take aspirin with food and not on an empty stomach. If you have to take it between meals, take it with a glass of milk. The buffering effect of milk is greater than any of the buffering agents sometimes combined with aspirin.

Often aspirin, or one of its derivatives, is combined with another painkiller, phenacetin, and with caffeine, which is a stimulant. Phenacetin is not dangerous when taken occasionally, but excessive and continued use could be toxic to the kidney. Phenacetin may also reduce the capacity of hemoglobin to carry oxygen by changing its form to methemoglobin. Never take phenacetin-containing pills in more than the recommended daily dose for longer than ten days without consulting a physician.

Caffeine stimulates the nervous system and the muscles and gives many people a lift. It is not a painkiller, but it works well (for some people) with painkillers like aspirin and phenacetin, although in such preparations the amount of caffeine would seem too small to give anyone a lift (15 to 30 mg caffeine compared to 100 to 150 mg in a cup of coffee or tea).

Cold remedies are designed to relieve the symptoms of a cold; each is directed to a different group of symptoms. The analgesics or painkillers ease the headache and muscle pain. The decongestants and antihistamines shrink the swollen mucous membranes and dry up the sinus, and the cough suppressants relieve coughing. There are cold tablets that combine all these remedies. We should remember that so far there is no cure for the cold. These remedies only relieve the symptoms to make the cold bearable. It is reasonable to take these medications to ease discomfort. But to help a cold run its course in the shortest time possible, we have to strengthen the body in its fight against the invading cold germs.

Get plenty of rest and adequate nutrition. Don't just take time off from work, but literally stay in bed for the first day or two, so that the body can channel all its energies to fighting the invading germs. It is also essential to eat a balanced diet and score well in each of the eight areas of our rating system. In addition, take plenty of fluids, preferably orange juice or vitaminized apple juice. Drink a small glass of either four times a day. That will provide you with added vitamin C to combat the infection.

Antacid preparations are sold for heartburn, gas, indigestion, and upset stomach. Antacids do neutralize the stomach acidity to some extent, because they are mildly alkaline. But they should not be used in excess or frequently.

An occasional discomfort due to high acidity may be relieved by one dose of antacid, which will neutralize the acids momentarily, although the stomach juices will soon redevelop their normal acidity. Frequent doses of antacids to neutralize or eliminate this acidity could have adverse effects on the normal digestive functions of the stomach.

An effective antacid will contain both magnesium and aluminum salts. (The first is slightly laxative and the second is slightly constipating so they balance each other.) Sodium bicarbonate (baking soda) is fast-acting but its effect does not last. If repeated too often, it could cause alkelosis (the opposite to acidosis, or too much acidity). And, if you are on a sodium-restricted diet, you may wish to avoid it as a source of sodium.

In addition, antacid preparations may contain gas-absorbing resins or activated charcoal and digestive enzymes like papain.

The value of any antacid preparation will have to be tested by you individually. Always consider it as a temporary measure to relieve occasional discomfort. If digestive problems are frequent, it is important to consult a physician.

In choosing a laxative, avoid fast-acting and strong ones. They cause sudden and extensive loss of water and other nutrients. It is preferable to take a mild laxative, even if it takes 24 hours to act. Mineral oil should be avoided since it interferes with absorption of the fat-soluble vitamins such as A, D, E, and K.

If you can tolerate roughage, resort to a bran cereal or baked product. It may be all you need. There are also bulk-forming preparations, such as methylcellulose tablets, which are available in the drug store.

Anti-diarrhea agents should be thought of as a short-term expedient until you can discuss the cause and treatment of diarrhea with your physician. Diarrhea can be dangerous, particularly with children, because in the course of an acute episode, the body loses large amounts of water and nutrients, sometimes causing severe dehydration and upsetting the nutritional balance of certain minerals in the body.

If you have to use an anti-diarrhea agent until you see a physician, try a preparation containing kaolin (a clay) or pectin (from fruit rinds). They absorb irritants like bacteria and toxins and eliminate them from the intestines. Their drawback is that they also absorb the helpful bacteria in the intestines. But these could be replenished by eating "natural yogurt" or tablet preparations containing the yogurt bacteria.

Obesity reduction aids are not that at all. The truth is that no drug preparation sold on prescription or over-the-counter will reduce anyone's weight. A program of caloric restriction and exercise is the only way to weight reduction. However, some products may help you restrict calories. Metrecal and similar products, for example, are in reality formulated foods with known caloric content and a balance of protein, carbohydrates, and fat and most vitamins and minerals. In cans (as a fluid) or packs (as cookies), they offer convenient, caloric-restricted meals. But they shouldn't be relied upon for all meals. Use them for two meals and eat real food in sensible quantities in the third meal. It is also advisable not to take them continuously for extended periods of time (say not more than 10 days out of every month), as they lack some nutrients.

Artificial sweeteners such as saccharin and cyclamate can be helpful in cutting down on calories if you have a sweet tooth. If they leave an after-taste, lower the quantity. You might have to adjust to partially sweetened beverages, but that's all to the good: how else are you going to get rid of your sweet tooth?

Other slimming preparations are of limited value. Some contain sugar, along with some vitamins and minerals, on the assumption that a bit of sugar immediately before mealtime will reduce your appetite. If it does, more power to you; just do not exceed the dose.

There are also methylcellulose tablets that swell in the intestine to give a feeling of bulk. This may help the bowel movement, but to have a full sensation you will need the bulk in the stomach, not in the intestine. It is said that when "slim was in" those models who looked as if they never ate a bite, never did. They chewed Kleenex to fill their stomachs and relied on black coffee and cigarettes to keep them moving. Needless to say, their careers were short-lived.

Mild appetite depressants sold over the counter are generally ineffective, and the prescription of amphetamines for weight loss is in disrepute. Diuretics do not reduce fat. They increase the flow of urine and the weight reduction that results is due mainly to loss of water, not fat. The side effects include loss of potassium and other minerals which could be dangerous unless the proper supplements are given.

Fattening products are nothing but formulated foods. Eat the same amount of real food and you'll be better off.

Many products in the drugstore are for external use and have no nutritional effect at all. We only mention them to say that a useful book for checking out non-prescription remedies is *The Medicine Show*, published by Consumers Union, Mount Vernon, New York, 1973.

Whether your problem is internal or external, don't diagnose and treat yourself. In this day and age, when health and medical services can be insured and made available through community clinics and health centers as well as doctors' practices, everyone should be able to consult a physician. Always seek a reliable source and be well informed. Never take chances with your health.

REMEMBER

A good NutriScore rating will give you good health. Everyone gets sick at one time or another and our bodies need extra nutrition, so check with your doctor about which pills affect what foods and how.

Women on the Pill have increased needs for certain nutrients. Increase your intake from NutriScore areas A to G to the levels of the pregnant and nursing women, but stay on guard against the foods in area H.

Over-the-counter drugs must be taken with care. They, too, affect your nutritional balance. Check with your doctor.

Chapter 19

Let Nutrition Help You Enrich Your Life

Have you ever witnessed a dramatic change in life style as the result of a change in eating patterns? The dreary fat friend who lost 25 pounds and won a tennis tournament! The sickly associate who put in a vegetable patch, ate his produce, and didn't miss a day's work all summer!

We all have illustrations from life to support the fact that what we eat affects what we do.

The true value of good nutrition lies not only in the use our body makes of food but beyond that in the use we make of the body. The well nourished person feels vital, energetic, ready to take life on and live it fully. While the malnourished body can't help responding with fatigue and depression and lassitude, the responses brought about by good nourishment are energetic and positive.

Take, for example, that basic instinct, sex. Psychological factors play a very large part in sexual activity, but nutrition has its role, too, in creating psychological readiness. Nobody can say with certainty how far our nutritional state affects the hormonal changes before, during, and after sexual activity; however, since every atom of the body depends on one nutrient or another there's probably some connection.

Little is known about what we need to do to prepare our bodies for healthful sexual activity. However, from existing knowledge, we can predict certain needs. For example, sexual intercourse requires the body to be flexible, robust, and fit. The value of exercise and adequate nutrition can not be denied. If you want to be active sexually, you should see to it that you score well nutritionally. You should also exercise for fit muscle tone using aerobic type and yoga exercises.

The secretion of fluids during sexual intercourse deprives the body of some water as well as small amounts of trace elements, sugars, and amino acids. These sex fluids are formed through rather complex chemical reactions, which require adequate reserves in the body of protein, carbohydrates, vitamins, and minerals. In addition, if the partners have had a drink or two before they engaged in sexual intercourse, they are likely to become dehydrated. Have two or more tall glasses or even a pitcher of fruit juice handy. There is a great deal of energy spent during sexual activity, particularly if it is prolonged over a period of time. Fruit juices compensate the body not only for water but also for energy. Have fruit juice or you may find it more romantic to have fruits, particularly those that are ready-to-eat such as grapes, orange sections, or halved peaches.

As for NutriScore, it's meant to make you happier, not unhappy. Try to eat the correct amounts from all the areas in the rating chart knowing that every aspect of your life will profit from your well-balanced diet. But don't attempt to go too fast. If you find that the sudden inclusion of many whole grains causes your family to suffer gas cramps, level out and build up gradually to the amount of whole grains you desire. A little advance warning is always welcome.

Also, not everything agrees with everybody. If certain foods are hard for you to digest, try cutting down on the amount you eat of any food that causes you any discomfort. Often you are able to tolerate small amounts.

Remember that exercise goes with good nutrition. Exercise helps the body burn the calories and utilize the nutrients you have carefully fed it. The better condition your body is in, the more completely and efficiently it can use its food, and the better yet its condition becomes. Build physical activity and recreation into your way of life. Walk to and from work or at least the last mile or kilometer of your journey. It shouldn't take more than 15 minutes or so and certainly most of us could afford that much time. Go for a walk on your lunch break. Practice your favorite sports regularly with friends or family. Exercise regularly, even if it means owning a dog to take out running every day.

We have inherited bodies that require exercising regularly. You will find that with regular exercise you will feel better, sleep more soundly, think more clearly, digest your food well, and maintain a healthy appetite without gaining weight.

Emotional and mental health are connected with nutrition, too. How often do we hear, "We've all been so nervous we couldn't eat a bite," or "I felt cranky from dieting or waiting too long for dinner." Those times when we're too knotted up to eat or are edgy because we haven't eaten should occur as seldom as possible. Eating, like sleeping, is necessary and important for our mental and emotional stability.

Are you the kind of person who works hard and plays hard? Remember that a stressful situation at work or at play can ruin your appetite, cause digestive problems, stomach or bowel complications. Even boredom can depress your mind and thereby your appetite. To counteract these states, we believe everyone should plan a period of relaxation and satisfying leisure each day. It should be a time when the problems of work are put out of your thoughts, a time when you pander only to your own mind and emotions by listening to music, bird-watching, baking, telephoning old friends, doing whatever pleases *you*. A relaxed person eats better and his body functions better. The person who eats well has resources for coping with the ever-changing emotional and mental demands of modern life.

The choice is yours. We believe you, too, can see the great importance of nutritious eating to your health and happiness. Products may change, science may make new discoveries, but the basic principle will remain the same: our bodies are nourished by what we feed them, and only the best is good enough.

Appendices

Appendix A—The Nutrient Content of Foods

Food Item	Chart Number	Measure		Weight	Moisture	Food Energy	Protein
				g	%	Cal	g
Almonds	A14	¼ cup	(50 mL)	35	5	212	6
Apple	D1	1 medium		150	85	70	tr.
Apple juice, vitamin C added	C1	½ cup	(125 mL)	124	88	60	tr.
Apple pie, see pies, apple							
Applesauce—sweetened	D1	½ cup	(125 mL)	128	76	115	tr.
—unsweetened	D1	½ cup	(125 mL)	122	88	50	tr.
Apple turnover*	H2	1 medium		84	35	265	2
Apricots—raw	D5	3 medium		114	85	55	1
—canned	D5	½ cup	(125 mL)	128	77	110	1
—dried	D5	5 med. halves		30	4	80	2
Asparagus, cooked or canned	E1	½ cup	(125 mL)	78	94	15	2
Avocado	C2	1 medium		284	74	370	5
Bacon—side	H3	3 slices		22	8	135	8
—Canadian or back	A17	4 slices		84	54	245	23
Banana	D2	1 medium		175	76	100	1
Beans—common, cooked	A1	½ cup	(125 mL)	90	69	105	7
—baked with weiners	A1	½ cup	(125 mL)	130	71	182	10
—baked with pork and tomato sauce	A1	½ cup	(125 mL)	128	71	155	8
—chick peas, cooked & canned	A1	½ cup	(125 mL)	125	11	110	6
—kidney, cooked	A1	½ cup	(125 mL)	128	76	115	8
—Lima, cooked	A1	½ cup	(125 mL)	85	71	95	7
—snap (green), cooked	F1	½ cup	(125 mL)	62	92	15	1
—soybeans, cooked	A1	½ cup	(125 mL)	90	74	120	10
—yellow, cooked	F1	½ cup	(125 mL)	62	93	15	1
Beef, cooked							
Ground beef, broiled, lean	A2	3 oz.		85	60	185	23
Ground beef, broiled, regular	A2	3 oz.		85	54	245	21
Rib roast	A2	3 oz.		85	40	375	17
Pot roast, chuck	A2	3 oz.		85	53	245	23

Fat	Saturated (Total)	Un-saturated		Carbohydrate	Calcium	Iron	Vitamin A Value	Thiamin	Riboflavin	Niacin	Ascorbic Acid
		Oleic	Lin-oleic								
g	g	g	g	g	mg	mg	I.U.	mg	mg	mg	mg
19	1	13	4	7	83	1.7	0	0.08	0.33	1.2	0
tr.	0	0	0	18	8	0.4	50	0.04	0.02	0.1	3
tr.	0	0	0	15	8	0.8	—	0.01	0.02	0.1	44
tr.	0	0	0	30	5	0.6	50	0.02	0.02	tr.	2
tr.	0	0	0	13	5	0.6	50	0.02	0.01	tr.	1
15	—	—	—	30	16	0.6	—	0.01	0.04	0.3	2
tr.	0	0	0	14	18	0.5	2890	0.03	0.04	0.7	10
tr.	0	0	0	28	14	0.4	2255	0.02	0.03	0.4	5
0	0	0	0	20	20	1.7	3300	tr.	0.05	1.0	4
tr.	0	0	0	2	15	0.4	655	0.12	0.13	1.0	19
37	7	17	5	13	22	1.3	630	0.24	0.43	3.5	30
12	5	6	2	2	3	0.8	0	0.12	0.08	1.2	0
15	4	8	tr.	11	16	—	0	0.68	0.11	4.4	0
tr.	0	0	0	26	10	0.8	230	0.06	0.07	0.8	12
tr.	0	0	0	19	45	2.5	0	0.13	0.07	0.7	0
9	—	—	—	16	47	2.4	165	0.09	0.08	1.7	tr.
4	1	1	tr.	25	69	2.3	165	0.10	0.04	0.8	3
1	0	tr.	tr.	18	45	2.1	15	0.10	0.03	0.6	0
tr.	0	0	0	21	37	2.3	5	0.07	0.05	0.8	—
tr.	0	0	0	17	40	2.1	240	0.16	0.09	1.1	15
tr.	0	0	0	4	32	0.4	340	0.04	0.06	0.3	8
5	1	1	3	10	65	2.5	20	0.20	0.08	0.6	0
tr.	0	0	0	3	32	0.4	145	0.04	0.06	0.3	8
10	5	4	tr.	0	10	3.0	20	0.08	0.20	5.1	0
17	8	8	tr.	0	9	2.7	30	0.07	0.18	4.6	0
34	16	15	1	0	8	2.2	70	0.05	0.13	3.1	0
16	8	7	tr.	0	10	2.9	30	0.04	0.18	3.5	0

Food Item	Chart Number	Measure		Weight g	Moisture %	Food Energy Cal	Protein g
Sirloin steak	A2	3 oz.		85	44	330	20
Round steak	A2	3 oz.		85	55	220	24
Beef and vegetable stew	A3	1 cup	(250 mL)	235	82	210	15
Beef pot pie	A3	1 pie		227	63	560	23
Beer	H1	12 fl. oz.	(375 mL)	360	92	150	1
Beets, cooked	F8	½ cup	(125 mL)	85	91	28	1
Biscuits (tea biscuits)	G12	1		28	27	105	2
Blackberries	C3	¾ cup	(175 mL)	108	84	64	2
Blueberries	C3	¾ cup	(175 mL)	105	83	64	1
Bologna	A13	2 slices		26	56	80	3
Bread and Buns							
Bagels	G1	half		30	—	90	3
Cornbread	G1	1 piece		30	51	100	2
Cracked wheat	G1	1 slice		25	35	65	2
French loaf	G1	1 slice		25	31	70	2
Raisin (18 slices per loaf)	G1	1 slice		25	35	65	2
Rye, light	G1	1 slice		30	35	73	3
Rye, dark, pumpernickel	G2	1 slice		32	34	79	3
White, enriched, 24 slices/loaf	G1	1 slice		30	35	82	2
Whole wheat	G2	1 slice		30	35	72	3
Breakfast cereals—dry, ready-to-eat							
Bran flakes, with added nutrients	G4	¾ cup	(175 mL)	28	3	104	3
Corn flakes, added nutrients	G4	1 cup	(250 mL)	21	4	80	2
Corn flakes, pre-sweetened, added nutrients	H6	1 cup	(250 mL)	28	2	107	1
Oats, puffed, with or without corn	G4	1 cup	(250 mL)	25	3	100	3
Oats, puffed, pre-sweetened	H6	¾ cup	(175 mL)	25	2	107	2
Rice, puffed or oven popped with added nutrients	G4	1 cup	(250 mL)	28	4	106	2

Fat	Saturated (Total)	Fatty Acids Unsaturated Oleic	Fatty Acids Unsaturated Linoleic	Carbohydrate	Calcium	Iron	Vitamin A Value	Thiamin	Riboflavin	Niacin	Ascorbic Acid
g	g	g	g	g	mg	mg	I.U.	mg	mg	mg	mg
27	13	12	1	0	9	2.5	50	0.05	0.16	4.0	0
13	6	6	tr.	0	10	3.0	20	0.07	0.19	4.8	0
10	5	4	tr.	15	28	2.8	2310	0.13	0.17	4.4	15
33	9	20	2	43	32	4.1	1860	0.25	0.27	4.5	7
0	0	0	0	14	18	tr.	—	0.01	0.11	2.2	0
tr.	0	0	0	6	12	0.4	15	0.02	0.04	0.2	5
5	1	2	1	13	34	0.4	tr.	0.06	0.06	0.1	—
1	0	0	0	14	34	0.9	217	0.04	0.04	0.4	22
1	0	0	0	16	16	1.0	105	0.03	0.06	0.4	15
7	—	—	—	tr.	2	0.5	—	0.04	0.06	0.7	—
1	0	tr.	tr.	15	5	0.7	tr.	0.08	0.06	0.7	0
3	0	tr.	1	16	75	0.4	80	0.06	0.06	0.4	0
1	0	0	tr.	13	20	0.3	tr.	0.03	0.02	0.3	0
1	0	0	tr.	14	10	0.6	0	0.07	0.06	0.6	0
tr.	0	0	0	13	18	0.3	0	0.01	0.02	0.2	—
tr.	0	0	0	16	22	0.5	0	0.05	0.02	0.4	0
tr.	0	0	0	17	27	0.8	0	0.07	0.04	0.4	0
1	0	0	0	15	20	0.5	0	0.07	0.05	0.7	0
1	0	0	0	15	15	0.7	0	0.05	0.03	1.0	0
tr.	0	0	0	22	13	4.0	0	0.60	1.00	6.0	0
tr.	0	0	0	18	1	3.0	0	0.45	0.75	4.5	0
tr.	0	0	0	25	1	4.0	0	0.60	0.80	6.0	0
1	0	0	0	25	23	1.0	0	0.02	—	0.5	0
1	0	0	0	25	23	1.0	0	0.03	0.03	0.4	0
tr.	0	0	0	24	5	4.0	0	0.60	1.00	6.0	0

Food Item	Chart Number	Measure		Weight	Moisture	Food Energy	Protein
				g	%	Cal	g
Rice, puffed or oven popped, presweetened with added nutrients	H6	1 cup	(250 mL)	28	4	120	1
Wheat flakes, with added nutrients	G4	1 cup	(250 mL)	28	4	105	3
Wheat puffed, presweetened with added nutrients	H6	1 cup	(250 mL)	21	3	80	1
Wheat, shredded 1 biscuit=12 spoon size	G6	1 biscuit		25	7	80	2
Wheat, shreaded, with added nutrients	G6	⅔ cup	(150 mL)	30	35	138	3
Farina, quick cooking, cooked: enriched	G3	1 cup	(250 mL)	245	89	105	3
Oatmeal or rolled oats, cooked	G5	1 cup	(250 mL)	240	87	130	5
Broccoli, cooked	E2	½ cup	(125 mL)	78	91	20	2
Brussels sprouts, cooked	E3	½ cup	(125 mL)	78	88	28	4
Butter	H4	1 tsp.	(5 mL)	5	16	35	tr.
Blended Butter	H4	1 tsp.	(5 mL)	5	15	35	0
Buttermilk	B4	1 cup	(250 mL)	245	90	90	9
Cabbage—raw	C4	½ cup	(125 mL)	45	92	10	1
—cooked	C4	½ cup	(125 mL)	85	94	18	1
Cabbage rolls, with meat	A4	2		206	55	261	9
Cakes							
Angelfood	H5	1 piece		53	34	135	3
Black Forest	H5	1 piece		90	21	310	4
Cheesecake	H5	1 piece		85	48	225	6
Cupcake, iced	H5	1 medium		50	22	190	2
Devil's Food	H5	1 piece		69	24	235	3
Gingerbread	H5	1 piece		65	31	170	2
White, without icing	H5	1 piece		86	25	315	4
White, with icing	H5	1 piece		114	23	400	4
Candy							
Gum drops	H7	1 oz.		28	12	100	tr.
Hard candy	H7	1 oz.		28	1	110	0

Fat	Saturated (Total)	Fatty Acids		Carbohydrate	Calcium	Iron	Vitamin A Value	Thiamin	Riboflavin	Niacin	Ascorbic Acid
		Un-saturated									
		Oleic	Lin-oleic								
g	g	g	g	g	mg	mg	I.U.	mg	mg	mg	mg
2	—	—	—	24	5	0.7	0	0.60	1.00	6.0	0
tr.	0	0	0	23	10	4.0	0	0.60	1.00	6.0	0
tr.	0	0	0	18	2	0.7	0	0.40	0.75	4.5	0
tr.	0	0	0	18	10	0.8	0	0.06	0.02	1.3	0
tr.	0	0	0	27	16	1.0	0	0.60	1.00	6.0	0
tr.	0	0	0	21	180	15.5	0	0.05	0.02	0.3	0
2	—	—	—	23	22	1.4	0	0.19	0.05	0.2	0
tr.	0	0	0	4	68	0.6	1940	0.07	0.15	0.6	70
tr.	0	0	0	5	25	.8	405	0.06	0.11	0.6	68
4	2	1	tr.	tr.	1	0	170	tr.	tr.	tr.	0
4	2	tr.	2	0	0	0	100	0	0	0	0
tr.	0	0	0	13	298	0.1	10	0.09	0.44	0.2	2
tr.	0	0	0	2	22	0.2	60	0.02	0.02	0.2	42
tr.	0	0	0	3	32	0.2	95	0.03	0.03	0.2	24
19	7	7	4	13	66	2.1	480	0.12	0.13	2.2	52
tr.	0	0	0	32	50	0.2	0	tr.	0.06	0.1	0
11	7	4	tr.	55	55	0.7	150	0.03	0.07	0.3	0
12	—	—	—	24	80	0.5	200	0.05	0.10	0.3	tr.
6	2	3	tr.	30	60	0.4	80	0.02	0.05	0.1	0
9	3	4	1	40	41	0.6	100	0.02	0.06	0.2	0
5	—	—	—	30	55	1.0	tr.	0.02	0.06	0.5	0
12	3	6	2	48	55	0.3	150	0.02	0.08	0.2	0
12	3	6	2	71	56	0.3	150	0.02	0.08	0.2	0
tr.	0	0	0	25	2	0.1	0	0	tr.	tr.	0
tr.	0	0	0	28	6	0.5	0	0	0	0	0

Food Item	Chart Number	Measure		Weight	Moisture	Food Energy	Protein
				g	%	Cal	g
Marshmallows	H7	1 oz.		28	17	90	1
Milk chocolate bars:							
All varieties	H7	1¼ oz.		35	8	168	3
"Caravan," "Caramilk" type	H7	1 oz.		30	8	116	1
"Oh Henry" type	H7	1 oz.		30	7	129	3
Cantaloupe	C5	¼		192	91	30	tr.
Carrots—raw	F2	1		50	88	20	1
—cooked	F2	½ cup	(125 mL)	72	91	22	tr.
Cashew nuts	A14	¼ cup	(50 mL)	35	5	196	6
Cauliflower, raw	C6	½ cup	(125 mL)	50	91	15	2
Cauliflower, cooked	C6	¾ cup	(175 mL)	110	93	24	2
Celery, raw	E4	1 stalk		40	94	5	tr.
Cereal—see Breakfast Cereals							
Cheeseburger—with bun							
A9 & B1 & G1		1		166	45	485	31
Cheeses							
Blue	B1	1 oz.		28	40	105	6
Camembert	B1	1 oz.		28	52	84	5
Cheddar (1" cube=17 gm.)	B1	1 oz.		28	37	116	7
Cheddar, processed	B1	1 oz.		28	40	105	7
Cottage, creamed (4% fat)	B2	½ cup	(125 mL)	113	79	120	16
Cottage, not creamed	B2	½ cup	(125 mL)	100	79	85	17
Cream	H4	1 oz./ 2 tbsp.	(25 mL)	28	i1	105	2
Swiss, processed, domestic	B1	1 oz.		28	40	100	8
Swiss, processed, gruyere	B1	1 oz.		28	40	115	8
Chelsea bun, cinnamon bun	H10	1		50	31	158	3
Cherries—raw	D5	½ cup	(125 mL)	80	80	59	1
—canned in syrup	D5	½ cup	(125 mL)	128	78	104	1
Chicken							
Breast, fried (½ breast) with bone	A5	3.3 oz.		95	58	155	25
Creamed	A5	½ cup	(125 ml)	120	68	210	18
Meat only (1 c. diced=5⅓ oz.)	A5	3 oz.		85	71	115	20
Roasted, skinned	A5	3½ oz.		100	54	170	32
Chicken pot pie	A5	1		227	63	535	23
Chili con carne—with beans	A1	½ cup	(125 mL)	125	72	168	10
—without beans	A1	½ cup	(125 mL)	128	67	255	13

Fat	Saturated (Total)	Fatty Acids Oleic	Un-saturated Lin-oleic	Carbohydrate	Calcium	Iron	Vitamin A Value	Thiamin	Riboflavin	Niacin	Ascorbic Acid
g	g	g	g	g	mg	mg	I.U.	mg	mg	mg	mg
tr.	0	0	0	23	5	0.5	0	0	tr.	tr.	0
8	5	3	tr.	22	31	0.9	tr.	0.02	0.06	2.0	0
4	2	2	tr.	20	36	0.4	10	0.02	0.05	tr.	tr.
6	2	3	1	16	36	0.3	tr.	0.07	0.04	1.0	tr.
tr.	0	0	0	7	14	0.4	3270	0.04	0.06	0.6	32
tr.	0	0	0	5	18	0.4	5500	0.03	0.03	0.3	4
tr.	0	0	0	5	24	0.4	7610	0.04	0.04	0.4	4
16	3	11	1	10	14	1.4	35	0.15	0.09	0.6	0
tr.	0	0	0	3	110	0.6	60	0.10	0.10	0.7	75
tr.	0	0	0	4	23	0.8	66	1.00	0.09	0.7	61
tr.	0	0	0	2	16	0.1	100	0.01	0.01	0.1	4
26	11	11	tr.	30	205	3.9	260	0.21	0.37	6.0	0
9	5	3	tr.	1	89	0.1	350	0.01	0.17	0.3	0
5	3	2	tr.	1	29	0.1	280	0.01	0.21	0.2	0
8	5	3	tr.	tr.	211	0.3	360	tr.	0.13	tr.	0
9	5	3	tr.	tr.	219	0.3	350	tr.	0.12	tr.	0
5	3	2	tr.	4	106	0.4	190	0.04	0.28	0.1	0
tr.	2	tr.	tr.	3	90	0.4	10	0.03	0.28	0.1	0
11	6	4	tr.	1	18	0.1	440	tr.	0.07	tr.	0
8	4	3	tr.	1	251	0.3	310	tr.	0.11	tr.	0
9	5	3	tr.	1	308	0.3	560	0	0.14	0.1	0
5	—	—	—	26	27	0.9	210	0.08	0.09	0.8	0
tr.	0	0	0	14	18	0.3	88	0.04	0.05	0.3	8
tr.	0	0	0	26	19	0.4	77	0.02	0.02	0.2	4
5	1	2	1	1	9	1.3	70	0.04	0.17	11.2	0
12	4	6	1	7	85	1.1	300	0.04	0.20	4.0	tr.
3	1	1	1	0	8	1.4	80	0.05	0.16	7.4	0
3	1	1	tr.	0	12	1.4	60	0.04	0.10	11.5	0
31	10	15	3	42	68	3.0	3020	0.25	0.26	4.1	5
8	4	4	tr.	15	40	2.1	75	0.04	0.09	1.6	0
19	9	9	tr.	8	49	1.8	190	0.03	0.16	2.8	0

Food Item	Chart Number	Measure		Weight	Moisture	Food Energy	Protein
				g	%	Cal	g
Chocolate bar—see Candy							
Chop suey, with meat	A6	1 cup	(250 mL)	250	75	300	26
Chow mein, with chicken	A6	1 cup	(250 mL)	220	78	224	27
Clams	A8	3 oz.		85	86	45	7
Coconut	A14	¼ cup	(50 mL)	15	4	86	tr.
Coffee with cream and sugar	H8	2 cups	(500 mL)	500	98	86	tr.
Coleslaw	F8	½ cup	(125 mL)	100	83	99	1
Cookies							
Brownies with nuts: (made from home recipe with enriched flour)	H5	1		20	10	95	1
Chocolate chip: (made from home recipe with enriched flour)	H10	1		10	3	50	1
Chocolate chip: commercial	H10	1		10	3	50	1
Chocolate marshmallow	H10	1		19	10	75	1
Fig bars, commercial	H10	1		14	14	50	1
Sandwich, chocolate or vanilla, commercial	H10	1		10	2	50	1
Social tea or Arrowroot	H10	1		5	2	20	tr.
Oatmeal, commercial	H10	1		19	3	86	1
Corn—whole cob	F8	1 ear		140	74	70	3
—kernels, cooked or canned	F8	½ cup	(125 mL)	83	79	70	2
Corn chips	H21	1-1½ cup	(250 mL -375 mL)	30	2	160	2
Corned beef	A2	3 oz.		85	59	185	22
Crab	A8	3oz.		85	77	85	15
Crackers							
Graham,	G8	4-2½" square	(4-6 cm square)	28	6	110	2
Saltines,	G7	4-2" square	(4-5 cm square)	11	4	50	1
Rye wafers	G8	4		28	6	96	4
Whole wheat	G8	4		28	7	113	2
Cream—light, for coffee	H4	1 tbsp	(15 mL)	15	72	30	1
—half & half	H4	1 tbsp		15	80	20	0.5
—heavy whipping	H4	1 tbsp		15	62	53	0.3
—sour	H4	1 tbsp		15	70	33	0.5

| | Fatty Acids | | | | | | | | | | |
Fat	Saturated (Total)	Oleic	Lin-oleic (Un-saturated)	Carbohydrate	Calcium	Iron	Vitamin A Value	Thiamin	Riboflavin	Niacin	Ascorbic Acid
g	g	g	g	g	mg	mg	I.U.	mg	mg	mg	mg
17	—	—	—	13	60	4.8	600	0.28	0.38	5.0	33
9	—	—	—	9	51	2.2	242	0.07	0.20	3.7	9
1	—	—	—	2	47	3.5	—	0.01	0.09	0.9	—
6	5	tr.	tr.	8	7	0.5	0	tr.	0.02	0.1	0
6	4	2	tr.	8	30	tr.	260	tr.	0.04	tr.	tr.
8	—	—	—	7	43	0.4	150	0.05	0.05	0.3	29
6	1	3	1	10	8	0.4	40	0.04	0.02	0.1	0
3	1	1	1	6	4	0.2	10	0.01	0.01	0.1	0
2	1	1	tr.	7	4	0.2	10	tr.	tr.	tr.	0
2	—	—	—	14	5	0.3	10	tr.	0.01	tr.	0
1	—	—	—	11	11	0.2	20	tr.	0.01	0.1	tr.
2	1	1	tr.	7	2	0.1	0	tr.	tr.	0.1	0
1	tr.	tr.	tr.	4	—	—	—	—	—	—	0
3	—	—	—	13	—	—	—	—	—	—	0
1	—	—	—	16	2	0.5	310	0.09	0.08	1.0	7
tr.	0	0	0	16	4	0.4	290	0.02	0.04	0.7	4
10	—	—	—	15	—	—	—	—	—	—	—
10	5	4	tr.	0	17	3.7	20	0.01	0.20	2.9	0
2	—	—	—	1	38	0.7	—	0.07	0.07	1.6	0
3	—	—	—	21	11	0.4	0	0.01	0.06	0.4	0
1	0	1	0	8	2	0.1	0	tr.	tr.	0.1	0
tr.	0	0	0	21	15	1.1	0	0.09	0.07	0.3	0
4	—	—	—	19	6	0.1	0	0.02	0.01	0.2	0
3	2	1	tr.	1	15	tr.	130	tr.	0.02	tr.	tr.
2	1	0.5	tr.	1	16	tr.	75	tr.	0.02	tr.	tr.
6	3	1	tr.	0.5	11	tr.	213	tr.	0.02	tr.	tr.
3	2	1	tr.	0.5	15	tr.	113	tr.	0.02	tr.	tr.

Food Item	Chart Number	Measure		Weight	Moisture	Food Energy	Protein
				g	%	Cal	g
Coffee whitener	H4	1 tsp		3	1	15	0
Non-dairy topping	H4	2 tbsp		10	50	30	0
Crisp, fruit	H5	1 piece		145	49	300	1
Cucumbers	E5	6 slices		50	96	5	tr.
Custard	B5	½ cup	(125 mL)	124	38	142	7
Danish pastry	H10	1		65	22	275	5
Dates	D3	1 oz.		30	22	77	1
Doughnuts	H10	1		32	24	125	1
Duck—see Goose							
Eclairs	H5	1		110	—	315	8
Eggs							
Boiled or poached	A7	1		50	74	80	6
Scrambled	A7	1		64	72	110	7
Fried	A7	1		55	70	113	6
Eggplant	F8	½ cup	(125 mL)	100	19	19	1
Eggroll	H11	1 medium		73	—	239	4
Farina (Wheatlets, Cream of Wheat)—see Breakfast Cereals							
Figs	D3	1 oz.		30	23	77	1
Fish—see also Salmon, Sardines and Tuna							
Cod, fried in butter	A8	4 oz.		95	65	162	26
Haddock, fried, breaded	A8	3 oz.		85	66	140	17
Halibut, grilled with butter	A8	3 oz.		85	67	146	21
Herring	A8	1 herring		85	63	217	17
Lobster, canned	A8	3 oz.		85	77	150	31
Mackerel, cooked	A8	3 oz.		85	62	200	19
Ocean perch, breaded, fried	A8	3 oz.		85	59	195	16
Sole—fillet, in butter	A8	3 oz.		85	58	172	26
Frankfurter	A19	1		56	57	170	7
French fries	H12	10		57	45	155	2
Fruit cocktail	D5	½ cup	(125 mL)	128	80	98	tr.
Fruit drinks with added vitamin C	H13	1 cup	(250 mL)	250	86	135	tr.
Fudge	H5	1½ oz.		42	8	116	2

| Fat | Saturated (Total) | Un-saturated | | Carbohydrate | Calcium | Iron | Vitamin A Value | Thiamin | Riboflavin | Niacin | Ascorbic Acid |
| | | Oleic | Linoleic | | | | | | | | |
g	g	g	g	g	mg	mg	I.U.	mg	mg	mg	mg
1	1	0	0	2	1	tr.	tr.	0	0	0	0
3	2	0	0	2	1	tr.	tr.	0	0	0	0
8	—	—	—	58	10	0.7	360	0.05	0.03	0.4	2
tr.	0	0	0	2	8	0.2	tr.	0.02	0.02	0.1	6
7	3	3	tr.	14	139	0.5	435	0.05	0.23	0.1	tr.
15	5	7	3	30	33	0.6	200	0.05	0.10	0.5	0
tr.	0	0	0	20	16	0.8	14	0.02	0.03	0.6	0
6	1	4	tr.	16	13	0.4	30	0.05	0.05	0.4	0
15	—	—	—	39	90	1.3	730	0.12	0.24	1.0	0
6	2	3	tr.	tr.	27	1.1	590	0.05	0.15	tr.	0
8	3	3	tr.	1	51	1.1	690	0.05	0.18	tr.	0
10	4	4	tr.	—	28	1.1	740	0.05	0.15	0	0
0	0	0	0	0	11	0.6	10	0.05	0.04	0.5	3
10	2	6	9	9	14	0.8	120	0.07	0.07	0.8	5
tr.	0	0	0	19	35	0.8	22	0.03	0.03	0.2	0
5	2	1	tr.	—	29	0.9	170	0.08	0.10	2.8	0
5	1	3	tr.	5	34	1.0	—	0.03	0.06	2.7	2
6	—	—	—	0	14	0.7	580	0.04	0.06	7.1	0
16	—	—	—	0	—	1.2	130	0.14	0.15	3.3	0
2	—	—	—	—	110	1.4	—	0.06	0.12	3.8	0
13	—	—	—	0	5	1.0	450	0.13	0.23	6.5	0
11	—	—	—	6	28	1.1	—	0.08	0.09	1.5	0
7	3	2	tr.	0	20	1.2	—	0.06	0.07	2.0	0
15	—	—	—	1	3	0.8	—	0.08	0.11	1.4	0
7	2	2	4	20	9	0.7	tr.	0.07	0.04	1.8	12
tr.	0	0	0	25	12	0.5	180	0.02	0.02	0.6	2
tr.	0	0	0	35	0	0	0	0	0	0	40
5	2	2	2	32	33	0.5	tr.	0.02	0.05	0.2	tr.

Food Item	Chart Number	Measure		Weight	Moisture	Food Energy	Protein
				g	%	Cal	g
Gelatin desserts	H14	¾ cup	(175 mL)	90	84	60	2
Goose or duck, cooked	A5	3 oz.		85	55	198	29
Grapefruit	C7	½		241	89	45	1
Grapefruit juice	C7	½ cup	(125 mL)	123	90	48	tr.
Grapes	D4	½ cup	(125 mL)	76	82	32	tr.
Grape juice	D4	½ cup	(125 mL)	126	83	82	tr.
Gravy	H4	2 tbsp		36	68	85	0
Ham	A17	3 oz.		85	54	245	18
Hamburger—with bun	A9 & G1	1 burger		145	46	409	25
Heart, beef	A12	2 oz.		57	41	107	18
Honey	H15	2 tbsp.	(25 mL)	42	34	130	tr.
Ice cream	H16	¾ cup	(175 mL)	100	63	191	4
Ice cream sundae	H17	1 cup	(250 mL)	204	64	336	7
Jams and preserves	H15	2 tbsp.	(25 mL)	40	58	110	tr.
Jellies	H15	2 tbsp.	(25 mL)	35	58	110	tr.
Kale, cooked	F3	½ cup	(125 mL)	90	91	25	3
Kidneys—beef	A12	2 oz.		57	53	103	11
—pork	A 12	2 oz.		57	55	65	9
Lamb, chop	A10	1, bone in		135	47	400	25
	A10	1, no bone		112	47	400	25
Lamb, leg roast	A10	3 oz.		85	54	235	22
Lasagna**—with meat	A11	1 cup	(250 mL)	384	69	538	38
—without meat	G9	½ cup	(125 mL)	170	70	208	14
Lentils, cooked	A1	½ cup	(125 mL)	75	69	80	6
Lettuce, leaves	E7	2 large		50	94	10	1
Lima Beans—see Beans							
Liver							
Beef liver, fried	A12	2 oz.		57	57	130	15
Calves liver, fried (2½" × 2¼" × ⅜") (6.25 × 5.5 × 1 cm)	A12	2 slices		58	52	118	13
Chicken liver, fried	A12	2 livers		60	65	148	18

Fat	Fatty Acids			Carbohydrate	Calcium	Iron	Vitamin A Value	Thiamin	Riboflavin	Niacin	Ascorbic Acid
	Saturated (Total)	Un-saturated									
		Oleic	Lin-oleic								
g	g	g	g	g	mg	mg	I.U.	mg	mg	mg	mg
0	0	0	0	14	0	0	0	0	0	0	0
8	—	—	—	0	12	1.4	—	0.09	0.14	7.9	0
tr.	0	0	0	12	19	0.5	10	0.05	0.02	0.2	44
tr.	0	0	0	12	11	0.2	10	0.04	0.02	0.2	46
tr.	0	0	0	8	8	0.2	50	0.02	0.02	0.1	2
tr.	0	0	0	21	14	0.4	—	0.05	0.02	0.2	20
7	—	—	—	4	0	0.2	0	0.02	0.01	0	0
19	7	8	2	0	8	2.2	0	0.40	0.16	3.1	0
19	8	9	tr.	30	49	3.7	30	0.21	0.28	6.0	0
3	—	—	—	1	3	3.0	13	0.14	0.07	4.4	1
0	—	—	—	34	2	0.2	0	tr.	0.02	0.2	tr.
10	6	4	tr.	21	146	0.1	442	0.04	0.21	0.1	1
8	12	10	6	59	268	1.5	582	0.14	0.39	0.7	1
tr.	0	0	0	28	8	0.4	tr.	tr.	0.02	tr.	tr.
tr.	0	0	0	26	8	0.6	tr.	tr.	0.02	tr.	1
1	—	—	—	4	121	1.1	6660	0.19	0.16	1.4	56
6	—	—	—	1	7	5.8	756	0.11	1.21	2.3	0
3	—	—	—	1	6	4.6	74	0.33	0.97	5.6	7
33	18	12	1	0	10	1.5	—	0.14	0.25	5.6	—
33	18	12	1	0	10	1.5	—	0.14	0.25	5.6	—
16	9	6	tr.	0	9	1.4	—	0.13	0.23	4.7	—
30	11	9	1	32	514	3.1	1980	0.13	0.52	3.6	20
11	4	3	1	16	255	0.9	983	0.05	0.22	0.7	10
tr.	0	0	0	15	19	1.6	15	0.06	0.05	0.5	0
tr.	0	0	0	2	34	0.7	950	0.03	0.04	0.2	9
6	—	—	—	3	6	5.0	30280	0.15	2.37	9.4	15
6	—	—	—	2	4	7.2	15300	0.10	1.90	9.4	21
7	—	—	—	2	—	6.0	25760	0.11	1.77	9.4	8

Food Item	Chart Number	Measure		Weight	Moisture	Food Energy	Protein
				g	%	Cal	g
Pork liver, fried (23½″ × 2¼″ × ⅜″) (6.25 × 5.5 × 1 cm)	A12	2 slices		59	54	136	14
Liver paste (paté)	A13	1 tbsp.	(15 mL)	15	37	70	2
Lobster—see Fish							
Lunch meats							
Bologna—see Bologna							
Salami—see Salami							
Canned lunch meat	A13	1 oz.		29	55	83	4
Macaroni, cooked	G9	½ cup	(125 mL)	70	72	78	3
Macaroni and cheese	B3	1 cup	(250 mL)	220	58	430	18
Mayonnaise	H4	1 tbsp.	(15 mL)	14	15	100	tr.
Milk							
Buttermilk	B4	1 cup	(250 mL)	245	91	90	9
Chocolate, low fat	B4	1 cup	(250 mL)	250	83	180	8
Evaporated	B4	½ cup	(125 mL)	125	74	170	9
Condensed, sweet	H4	2 tbsp.	(30 mL)	40	27	120	3
Human milk	B4	1 cup	(250 mL)	240	85	170	2
Whole, 3.5% fat	B4	1 cup	(250 mL)	244	87	160	9
Non fat (skim)	B4	1 cup	(250 mL)	245	90	90	9
Partially skimmed, 2% fat	B4	1 cup	(250 mL)	245	87	123	9
Milkshake	H17	1 cup	(250 mL)	270	83	280	13
Mixed vegetables	F4	½ cup	(125 mL)	80	83	51	2
Molasses—light (first extraction)	H15	1 tbsp.	(15 mL)	20	24	50	0
—blackstrap	H15	1 tbsp.	(15 mL)	20	24	45	0
Muffins—bran	G11	1		35	35	86	3
—plain	G10	1		40	38	120	3
—cornmeal	G10	1		40	33	125	3
Mushrooms, fresh, sauteed	F8	4 average		70	93	78	2
Nectarines	D5	1 medium		150	82	96	1
Noodles, cooked	G9	½ cup	(125 mL)	80	70	100	4
Nuts—see individual varieties by name, peanuts, etc.							
Onions—raw	F8	1		110	89	40	2
—cooked	F8	½ cup	(125 mL)	105	92	30	2

Fat	Fatty Acids Saturated (Total)	Un-saturated Oleic	Un-saturated Lin-oleic	Carbohydrate	Calcium	Iron	Vitamin A Value	Thiamin	Riboflavin	Niacin	Ascorbic Acid
g	g	g	g	g	mg	mg	I.U.	mg	mg	mg	mg
6	—	—	—	6	8	12.5	9660	0.20	1.84	9.9	8
7	—	—	—	1	0	0.5	1200	0.01	0.05	0.4	0
7	3	3	1	1	3	0.6	0	0.09	0.06	0.8	—
1	0	tr.	tr.	16	6	0.3	0	0.01	0.01	0.2	0
24	11	10	1	44	398	2.0	950	0.22	0.44	2.0	tr.
11	2	2	6	tr.	3	0.1	40	tr.	0.01	tr.	0
tr.	0	0	0	12	300	0.1	500	0.09	0.40	0.2	2
5	2	2	tr.	26	285	0.6	500	0.10	0.40	0.3	2
10	5	2	tr.	13	330	0.2	300	0.05	0.40	0.3	1
4	2	1	tr.	20	105	0.1	100	0.03	0.20	0.1	tr.
10	5	2	tr.	17	80	0.1	560	0.03	0.08	0.8	16
9	5	3	tr.	12	288	0.1	350	0.07	0.41	0.2	2
tr.	0	0	0	13	298	0.1	10	0.10	0.44	0.2	2
5	3	2	tr.	12	294	0.1	172	0.10	0.44	0.2	2
12	—	—	—	32	364	0.8	670	0.17	0.56	0.2	2
tr.	0	0	0	11	20	1.0	3960	0.10	0.06	0.9	6
0	0	0	0	13	33	0.9	0	0.01	0.01	tr.	0
0	0	0	0	11	137	3.2	0	0.02	0.04	0.4	0
3	tr.	2	tr.	14	35	1.3	60	0.07	0.09	1.5	0
4	1	2	1	17	42	0.6	40	0.07	0.09	0.6	tr.
4	1	2	1	20	96	0.6	100	0.07	0.08	0.6	0
7	3	2	tr.	3	8	0.7	170	0.05	0.28	2.9	tr.
tr.	0	0	0	26	6	0.8	2475	—	—	—	20
1	1	1	tr.	19	8	0.5	55	0.03	0.02	0.3	0
tr.	0	0	0	10	30	0.6	40	0.04	0.04	0.2	11
tr.	0	0	0	7	25	0.4	40	0.03	0.03	0.2	7

Food Item	Chart Number	Measure		Weight	Moisture	Food Energy	Protein
				g	%	Cal	g
Onions, french fried— see French fries							
Orange	C8	1		180	86	65	1
Orange juice	C8	½ cup	(125 mL)	124	88	55	1
Oysters	A8	3 oz.		85	82	65	7
Pancakes, plain	G12	1 (6" or 15 cm diam.)		40	50	90	3
with butter and syrup	H18	1 (6" or 15 cm diam.)		96	—	310	3
Parsley	E8	½ cup	(125 mL)	32	85	tr.	tr.
Parsnips, cooked	F8	⅓ cup	(80 mL)	78	82	50	1
Peaches, raw	D5	1		114	89	35	1
canned, in syrup	D5	½ cup	(125 mL)	128	79	100	tr.
Peanuts	A14	¼ cup	(50 mL)	36	2	210	9
Peanut butter	A15	2 tbsp.	(25 mL)	32	2	190	8
Pear, raw	D5	1		182	83	100	1
canned	D5	½ cup	(125 mL)	128	80	98	tr.
Peas, cooked	F4	½ cup	(125 mL)	80	82	58	4
dried, cooked	A1	½ cup	(125 mL)	125	70	145	10
Peppers, raw	C9	1 pod		74	93	15	1
cooked	C9	1 pod		73	95	15	1
Pies, apple	H19	1 sector		160	—	410	3
cherry	H19	1 sector		160	—	387	4
custard	H19	1 sector		150	58	327	9
lemon meringue	H19	1 sector		140	47	357	5
Pineapple, raw	D5	½ cup	(125 mL)	70	85	38	tr.
canned in syrup	D5	½ cup	(125 mL)	130	80	98	tr.
Pizza, cheese only	G9	1-5½" (14 cm) sector		75	45	185	7
sausage and cheese	A16	1-5½" (14 cm) sector		105	45	315	14
Plums, raw	D5	1		60	87	25	tr.
canned	D5	½ cup	(125 mL)	128	77	102	tr.
Popcorn, plain	H20	2 cups	(500 mL)	18	6	80	2
butter and salt	H20	2 cups	(500 mL)	28	—	150	2
Popsicle	H22	1		95	80	70	1

Fat	Fatty Acids			Carbohydrate	Calcium	Iron	Vitamin A Value	Thiamin	Riboflavin	Niacin	Ascorbic Acid
	Saturated (Total)	Unsaturated									
		Oleic	Linoleic								
g	g	g	g	g	mg	mg	I.U.	mg	mg	mg	mg
tr.	0	0	0	16	54	0.5	260	0.13	0.05	0.5	66
tr.	0	0	0	13	14	0.2	250	0.11	0.04	0.5	62
2	—	—	—	4	24	4.8	—	0.02	0.17	0.7	—
3	2	2	tr.	9	87	0.4	105	0.06	0.09	0.3	—
15	8	6	tr.	39	108	2.0	575	0.06	0.09	0.3	—
tr.	0	0	0	tr.	64	1.6	2720	tr.	0.08	tr.	56
tr.	0	0	0	12	35	0.4	25	0.06	0.06	0.1	8
tr.	0	0	0	10	9	0.5	1320	0.02	0.05	1.0	7
tr.	0	0	0	26	5	0.4	550	0.01	0.03	0.7	4
18	4	8	5	7	27	0.8	—	0.12	0.05	6.2	0
16	4	8	4	6	18	0.6	—	0.04	0.04	4.8	0
1	—	—	—	25	13	0.5	30	0.04	0.07	0.2	7
tr.	0	0	0	25	6	0.2	tr.	0.02	0.02	0.2	2
tr.	0	0	0	10	18	1.4	430	0.22	0.08	1.8	16
1	—	—	—	26	14	2.1	50	0.19	0.11	1.1	0
tr.	0	0	0	4	7	0.5	310	0.06	0.06	0.4	94
tr.	0	0	0	3	7	0.4	310	0.05	0.05	0.4	70
18	5	11	1	61	1	0.5	50	0.03	0.03	0.6	2
18	5	11	1	62	22	0.5	710	0.03	0.03	0.8	tr.
17	6	10	1	35	144	0.9	350	0.08	0.24	0.4	0
14	5	8	1	53	20	0.7	240	0.05	0.11	0.3	4
tr.	0	0	0	10	12	0.4	50	0.02	0.02	0.2	12
tr.	0	0	0	25	15	0.4	60	0.10	0.03	0.2	8
6	2	3	tr.	27	107	0.7	290	0.04	0.12	0.7	4
17	2	3	tr.	27	111	1.8	290	0.12	0.18	1.6	4
tr.	0	0	0	7	7	0.3	140	0.02	0.02	0.3	3
tr.	0	0	0	26	11	1.1	1485	0.02	0.02	0.4	2
4	2	tr.	tr.	10	2	0.4	—	—	0.02	0.2	0
12	6	2	tr.	10	4	0.4	340	—	0.02	0.2	0
tr.	0	0	0	17	tr.	tr.	0	tr.	tr.	tr.	—

Food Item	Chart Number	Measure		Weight	Moisture	Food Energy	Protein
				g	%	Cal	g
Pork, chop	A17	1		98	42	260	16
roast	A17	3 oz.		85	46	310	21
Potatoes, boiled	F5	1		122	83	80	2
baked	F5	1		99	75	90	3
fried-see French fries							
mashed	F5	½ cup	(125 mL)	98	80	93	2
scalloped, with cheese	F5	¼ cup	(60 mL)	60	71	88	3
hashed brown	F5	¼ cup	(60 mL)	50	54	115	2
Potato chips	H21	1 cup	(250 mL)	40	2	230	2
Prunes	D3	4		32	28	70	1
Pudding, instant	B5	½ cup	(125 mL)	157	66	182	6
rice	B5	½ cup	(125 mL)	97	67	141	3
tapioca	B5	½ cup	(125 mL)	105	70	133	5
Radishes	F8	4		40	94	5	tr.
Raisins	D3	1 oz.		28	18	80	tr.
Raspberries	C3	¾ cup	(175 mL)	92	84	52	tr.
Rhubarb, cooked	D5	½ cup	(125 mL)	136	63	192	tr.
Rice, regular or instant	G14	½ cup	(125 mL)	80	73	92	2
brown, parboiled or							
converted	G13	½ cup	(125 mL)	80	71	99	2
Rolls and buns							
white dinner roll	G10	1		30	40	90	2
hamburg or hot dog bun	G10	1		60	31	164	4
whole wheat roll	G11	1		30	40	79	3
Rye Krisp crackers—see Crackers, rye wafers							
Salami, dry	A13	1 oz.		28	30	130	7
cooked	A13	1 oz.		28	51	90	5
Salmon, canned, solids and liquids	B6	3 oz.		85	71	130	18
fresh, baked or broiled	B6	3 oz.		85	71	155	23
Sardines	A18	3 oz		85	62	175	20
Sausages	A19	3 links		39	35	188	8
Shrimp	A8	⅔ cup	(150 mL)	85	70	100	21
Soda crackers—see Crackers, saltines							

Fat	Saturated (Total)	Fatty Acids		Carbohydrate	Calcium	Iron	Vitamin A Value	Thiamin	Riboflavin	Niacin	Ascorbic Acid
		Un-saturated									
		Oleic	Lin-oleic								
g	g	g	g	g	mg	mg	I.U.	mg	mg	mg	mg
21	8	9	2	0	8	2.2	0	0.63	0.18	3.8	—
24	9	10	2	0	9	2.7	0	0.78	0.22	4.7	—
tr.	0	0	0	18	7	0.6	tr.	0.11	0.04	1.4	20
tr.	0	0	0	21	9	0.7	tr.	0.10	0.04	1.7	20
4	2	2	tr.	12	24	0.4	165	0.08	0.05	1.0	9
5	3	2	tr.	8	78	0.3	195	0.04	0.08	0.6	6
6	1	3	tr.	15	6	0.5	tr.	0.04	0.03	1.1	5
16	10	4	tr.	20	16	0.8	tr.	0.08	0.02	2.0	6
tr.	0	0	0	18	14	1.1	440	0.02	0.04	0.4	1
5	3	2	tr.	32	150	0.5	180	0.05	0.23	0.1	1
3	—	—	—	26	95	0.4	110	0.03	0.13	0.2	tr.
5	—	—	—	17	105	0.5	310	0.05	0.19	0.1	1
tr.	0	0	0	1	12	0.4	tr.	0.01	0.01	0.1	10
tr.	0	0	0	22	18	1.0	tr.	0.04	0.02	0.2	tr.
tr.	0	0	0	13	20	0.8	120	0.03	0.08	0.8	23
tr.	0	0	0	49	106	0.8	110	0.03	0.08	0.4	8
tr.	0	0	0	20	16	0.7	0	0.10	0.01	1.0	0
tr.	0	0	0	21	9	0.4	0	0.10	0.01	1.3	0
2	—	—	—	16	18	0.4	0	0.08	0.04	0.8	0
2	tr.	1	tr.	30	40	1.0	0	0.14	0.10	1.4	0
2	—	—	—	16	13	0.5	0	0.06	0.02	0.9	0
11	—	—	—	tr.	4	1.0	—	0.10	0.07	1.5	0
7	—	—	—	tr.	3	0.7	—	0.07	0.07	1.2	0
6	1	1	tr.	0	167	0.7	60	0.03	0.16	6.8	0
6	1	1	tr.	0	—	1.0	140	0.14	0.05	6.2	0
9	—	—	—	0	372	2.5	190	0.02	0.17	4.6	0
16	6	8	2	tr.	3	0.9	0	0.32	0.14	1.5	0
1	0	tr.	tr.	1	98	2.6	50	0.01	0.03	1.5	0

Food Item	Chart Number	Measure		Weight	Moisture	Food Energy	Protein
				g	%	Cal	g
Soft drinks, cola	H22	10 fl. oz.	(300 mL)	308	90	121	0
ginger ale	H22	10 fl. oz.	(300 mL)	305	92	95	0
Soups, made with milk							
Cream of chicken	B7	¾ cup	(175 mL)	138	85	101	4
Cream of mushroom	B7	¾ cup	(175 mL)	138	83	121	4
Cream of tomato	B7	¾ cup	(175 mL)	141	84	98	4
Spaghetti, cooked	G9	½ cup	(125 mL)	70	72	78	3
Spaghetti and meat sauce	A11	1 cup	(250 mL)	248	70	330	19
Spaghetti and tomato sauce	G9	½ cup	(125 mL)	125	80	145	3
Spinach	E6	½ cup	(125 mL)	90	92	20	2
Squash, summer	F7	½ cup	(125 mL)	105	96	15	1
winter	F6	½ cup	(125 mL)	102	81	65	2
Strawberries	C3	¾ cup	(175 mL)	112	90	41	tr.
Sugar	H15	1 tbsp.	(15 mL)	11	tr.	40	0
Sundae—see Ice cream sundae							
Sweet Potatoes	F6	1		110	64	155	2
Syrups, table blend	H15	1 tbsp.	(15 mL)	21	24	60	0
maple	H15	1 tbsp.	(15 mL)	21	—	50	0
Tangerines	C10	1		116	87	40	1
Tangerine juice	C10	½ cup	(125 mL)	124	88	58	tr.
Tapioca pudding—see Pudding							
Tea with cream and sugar	H8	2 cups	(500 mL)	500	98	86	2
Tomatoes, raw	C11	1 medium		150	94	35	2
canned	C11	¾ cup	(175 mL)	181	94	38	2
juice	C11	¾ cup	(175 mL)	182	94	34	2
Tongue, beef	A13	1 oz.		28	61	69	6
Tuna, canned in oil,							
solids only	A8	3 oz.		85	61	170	24
Tuna, canned in water,							
solids and liquids	A8	3 oz.		85	70	108	24
Turkey	A5	3 oz.		85	56	160	25
Turkey pot pie—see Chicken pot pie							
Turnips, cooked	F7	½ cup	(125 mL)	100	91	35	1
Turnover—see apple turnover							
Veal, cutlet	A2	3 oz.		85	60	185	23
roast	A2	3 oz.		85	55	230	23

Fat	Fatty Acids			Carbohydrate	Calcium	Iron	Vitamin A Value	Thiamin	Riboflavin	Niacin	Ascorbic Acid
	Saturated (Total)	Un-saturated									
		Oleic	Linoleic								
g	g	g	g	g	mg	mg	I.U.	mg	mg	mg	mg
0	0	0	0	31	—	—	0	0	0	0	0
0	0	0	0	24	—	—	0	0	0	0	0
8	2	2	3	9	107	0.3	141	0.03	0.17	0.4	1
6	2	2	2	8	97	0.3	344	0.03	0.15	0.4	2
4	2	2	1	13	95	0.5	675	0.06	0.14	0.8	8
1	0	tr.	tr.	16	6	0.3	0	0.01	0.01	0.2	0
12	4	6	1	39	125	3.8	1600	0.26	0.30	4.0	22
1	1	1	1	19	20	1.4	465	0.18	0.14	2.3	5
tr.	0	0	0	3	84	2.0	7290	0.06	0.12	0.5	25
tr.	0	0	0	4	26	0.4	410	0.05	0.08	0.8	10
tr.	0	0	0	16	28	0.8	4305	0.05	0.14	0.7	14
tr.	0	0	0	10	23	1.1	68	0.03	0.08	0.8	66
0	0	0	0	11	0	tr.	0	0	0	0	0
1	0	tr.	tr.	36	44	1.0	8910	0.10	0.07	0.7	24
0	0	0	0	15	9	0.8	0	0	0	0	0
0	0	0	0	13	33	0.6	0	0	0	0	0
tr.	0	0	0	10	34	0.3	360	0.05	0.02	0.1	27
tr.	0	0	0	14	22	0.2	510	0.07	0.02	0.2	34
6	4	2	tr.	10	30	tr.	260	tr.	0.04	tr.	tr.
tr.	0	0	0	7	20	0.8	1350	0.10	0.06	1.0	34
tr.	0	0	0	8	10	0.9	1628	0.09	0.05	1.3	31
tr.	0	0	0	8	13	1.6	1455	0.10	0.05	1.4	29
5	—	—	—	tr.	2	0.6	—	0.01	0.08	1.0	0
7	2	1	1	0	7	1.6	70	0.04	0.10	10.1	0
1	—	—	—	0	14	1.4	—	0.04	0.10	11.3	0
6	—	—	—	0	24	5.0	10	0.06	0.14	5.8	0
tr.	—	—	—	8	59	tr.	550	0.06	0.06	0.5	26
9	5	4	tr.	—	9	2.7	—	0.06	0.21	4.6	—
14	7	6	tr.	0	10	2.9	—	0.11	0.26	6.6	—

Food Item	Chart Number	Measure		Weight	Moisture	Food Energy	Protein
				g	%	Cal	g
Waffles, plain	G12	1 (6″ or 15 cm diam.)		64	41	180	6
with butter and syrup	H18	1 (6″ or 15 cm diam.)		120	32	400	6
Walnuts	A14	¼ cup	(50 mL)	25	4	162	4
Watermelon	D5	1 wedge		925	93	115	2
Weiners—see Frankfurters							
Wheat Bran	G15	3 tbsp.	(50 mL)	25	12	53	4
Wheat Germ	G15	3 tbsp.	(50 mL)	25	12	90	7
Wine, dessert	H1	5 fl. oz.	(150 mL)	140	77	196	—
table	H1	5 fl. oz.	(150 mL)	140	86	122	—
Yogurt, made from partially skimmed milk, plain	B8	6 oz.	(175 mL)	185	89	112	9
made from partially skimmed milk, fruit flavored (average)	B8	6 oz.	(175 mL)	185	89	170	8

Sources
 *Manufacturer's Data
**Calculated from Recipe

Fat	Saturated (Total)	Fatty Acids		Carbohydrate	Calcium	Iron	Vitamin A Value	Thiamin	Riboflavin	Niacin	Ascorbic Acid
		Oleic	Un-saturated Linoleic								
g	g	g	g	g	mg	mg	I.U.	mg	mg	mg	mg
6	2	3	1	24	73	1.1	214	0.11	0.16	0.8	0
18	8	7	1	54	94	2.7	684	0.11	0.16	0.8	0
16	1	2	10	4	25	0.8	8	0.08	0.03	0.2	—
1	—	—	—	27	30	2.1	2510	0.13	0.13	0.7	30
1	—	—	—	15	30	3.7	—	0.18	0.09	5.0	—
3	1	—	2	12	18	2.6	—	0.50	0.17	1.1	—
—	—	—	—	12	12	—	—	0.02	0.03	0.3	—
—	—	—	—	6	12	—	—	tr.	0.02	0.2	—
3	2	1	tr.	13	310	0.1	130	0.08	0.45	0.2	2
3	2	1	tr.	30	230	0.1	100	0.07	0.32	0.2	2

Sources:
1. Nutrient Value of Some Common Foods, Health and Welfare Canada, Ottawa, 1971.
2. Watt, B.K. and A.L. Merrill, Composition of Foods, Agriculture Handbook No. 8, U.S. Department of Agriculture, Washington, D.C., 1963.

Appendix B—Recommended Daily
Dietary Allowances—U.S.A.

Mean Heights and Weights and Recommended Energy Intake

Category	Age (years)	Weight (kg)	Weight (lb)	Height (cm)	Height (in)	Energy Needs (with range) (kcal)	(MJ)
Infants	0.0-0.5	6	13	60	24	kg X 115 (95-145)	kg X .48
	0.5-1.0	9	20	71	28	kg X 105 (80-135)	kg X .44
Children	1-3	13	29	90	35	1300 (900-1800)	5.5
	4-6	20	44	112	44	1700 (1300-2300)	7.1
	7-10	28	62	132	52	2400 (1650-3300)	10.1
Males	11-14	45	99	157	62	2700 (2000-3700)	11.3
	15-18	66	145	176	69	2800 (2100-3900)	11.8
	19-22	70	154	177	70	2900 (2500-3300)	12.2
	23-50	70	154	178	70	2700 (2300-3100)	11.3
	51-75	70	154	178	70	2400 (2000-2800)	10.1
	76+	70	154	178	70	2050 (1650-2450)	8.6
Females	11-14	46	101	157	62	2200 (1500-3000)	9.2
	15-18	55	120	163	64	2100 (1200-3000)	8.8
	19-22	55	120	163	64	2100 (1700-2500)	8.8
	23-50	55	120	163	64	2000 (1600-2400)	8.4
	51-75	55	120	163	64	1800 (1400-2200)	7.6
	76+	55	120	163	64	1600 (1200-2000)	6.7
Pregnancy						+ 300	
Lactation						+ 500	

The data in this table have been assembled from the observed median heights and weights of children shown in Table 1, together with desirable weights for adults given in Table 2 for the mean heights of men (70 inches or 178 cm) and women (64 inches or 163 cm) between the ages of 18 and 34 years as surveyed in the U.S. population (HEW/NCHS data).

The energy allowances for the young adults are for men and women doing light work. The allowances for the two older age groups represent mean energy needs over these age spans, allowing for a 2% decrease in basal (resting) metabolic rate per decade and a reduction in activity of 200 kcal/day for men and women between 51 and 75 years, 500 kcal for men over 75 years and 400 kcal for women over 75 (see text). The customary range of daily energy output is shown for adults in parentheses, and is based on a variation in energy needs of 400 kcal at any one age (see text and Garrow, 1978), emphasizing the wide range of energy intakes appropriate for any group of people.

Energy allowances for children through age 18 are based on median energy intakes of children these ages followed in longitudinal growth studies. The values in parentheses are 10th and 90th percentiles of energy intake, to indicate the range of energy consumption among children of these ages (see text).

From: Recommended Dietary Allowances, Revised 1979. Food and Nutrition Board National Academy of Sciences-National Research Council, Washington, D.C.

Estimated Safe and Adequate Daily Dietary Intakes of Additional Selected Vitamins and Minerals[a]

| | Vitamins | | | Trace Elements[b] | | | | | | Electrolytes | | |
Age (years)	Vitamin K (µg)	Biotin (µg)	Pantothenic Acid (mg)	Copper (mg)	Manganese (mg)	Fluoride (mg)	Chromium (mg)	Selenium (mg)	Molybdenum (mg)	Sodium (mg)	Potassium (mg)	Chloride (mg)
Infants 0-0.5	12	35	2	0.5-0.7	0.5-0.7	0.1-0.5	0.01-0.04	0.01-0.04	0.03-0.06	115-350	350-925	275-700
0.5-1	10-20	50	3	0.7-1.0	0.7-1.0	0.2-1.0	0.02-0.06	0.02-0.06	0.04-0.08	250-750	425-1275	400-1200
Children 1-3	15-30	65	3	1.0-1.5	1.0-1.5	0.5-1.5	0.02-0.08	0.02-0.08	0.05-0.1	325-975	550-1650	500-1500
and 4-6	20-40	85	3-4	1.5-2.0	1.5-2.0	1.0-2.5	0.03-0.12	0.03-0.12	0.06-0.15	450-1350	750-2325	700-2100
Adolescents 7-10	30-60	120	4-5	2.0-2.5	2.0-3.0	1.5-2.5	0.05-0.2	0.05-0.2	0.1-0.3	600-1800	1000-3000	925-2775
11+	50-100	100-200	4-7	2.0-3.0	2.5-5.0	1.5-2.5	0.05-0.2	0.05-0.2	0.15-0.5	900-2700	1525-4575	1400-4200
Adults	70-140	100-200	4-7	2.0-3.0	2.5-5.0	1.5-4.0	0.05-0.2	0.05-0.2	0.15-0.5	1100-3300	1875-5625	1700-5100

[a]Because there is less information on which to base allowances, these figures are not given in the main table of the RDA and are provided here in the form of ranges of recommended intakes.

[b]Since the toxic levels for many trace elements may be only several times usual intakes, the upper levels for the trace elements given in this table should not be habitually exceeded.

From: Recommended Dietary Allowances, Revised 1979. Food and Nutrition Board National Academy of Sciences–National Research Council, Washington, D.C.

243

Appendix C—Recommended Daily Intakes—
The Canadian Dietary Standard

Age	Sex	Weight	Height	Energy[a]	Protein	Thiamin	Niacin[e]	Riboflavin	Vitamin B₆f
yrs		kg	cm	kcal	gm	mg	mg	mg	mg
0-6 mo.	Both	6	—	kgx117	kgx2.2 (2.0)[d]	0.3	5	0.4	0.3
7-11 mo.	Both	9	—	kgx108	kgx1.4	0.5	6	0.6	0.4
1-3	Both	13	90	1,400	22	0.7	9	0.8	0.8
4-6	Both	19	110	1,800	27	0.9	12	1.1	1.3
7-9	M	27	129	2,200	33	1.1	14	1.3	1.6
	F	27	128	2,000	33	1.0	13	1.2	1.4
10-12	M	36	144	2,500	41	1.2	17	1.5	1.8
	F	38	145	2,300	40	1.1	15	1.4	1.5
13-15	M	51	162	2,800	52	1.4	19	1.7	2.0
	F	49	159	2,200	43	1.1	15	1.4	1.5
16-18	M	64	172	3,200	54	1.6	21	2.0	2.0
	F	54	161	2,100	43	1.1	14	1.3	1.5
19-35	M	70	176	3,000	56	1.5	20	1.8	2.0
	F	56	161	2,100	41	1.1	14	1.3	1.5

Folate[g]	Vitamin B$_{12}$	Ascorbic Acid	Vitamin A	Vitamin D	Vitamin E[j]	Calcium	Phosphorus	Magnesium	Iodine	Iron	Zinc
mcg	mcg	mg	mcg RE[i]	mcg[j]	mg[j]	mg	mg	mg	mcg	mg	mg
40	0.3	20[h]	400	10	3	500	250[l]	50[l]	35[l]	7[l]	4
60	0.3	20	400	10	3	500	400	50	50	7	5
100	0.9	20	400	10	4	500	500	75	70	8	5
100	1.5	20	500	5	5	500	500	100	90	9	6
100	1.5	30	700	2.5[k]	6	700	700	150	110	10	7
100	1.5	30	700	2.5[k]	6	700	700	150	100	10	.7
100	3.0	30	800	2.5[k]	7	900	900	175	130	11	8
100	3.0	30	800	2.5[k]	7	1,000	1,000	200	120	11	9
200	3.0	30	1,000	2.5[k]	9	1,200	1,200	250	140	13	10
200	3.0	30	800	2.5[k]	7	800	800	250	110	14	10
200	3.0	30	1,000	2.5[k]	10	1,000	1,000	300	160	14	12
200	3.0	30	800	2.5[k]	6	700	700	250	110	14	11
200	3.0	30	1,000	2.5[k]	9	800	800	300	150	10	10
200	3.0	30	800	2.5[k]	6	700	700	250	110	14	9

Age	Sex	Weight	Height	Energy[a]	Protein	Thiamin	Niacin[e]	Riboflavin	Vitamin B[f]
yrs		kg	cm	kcal	gm	mg	mg	mg	mg
36-50	M	70	176	2,700	56	1.4	18	1.7	2.0
	F	56	161	1,900	41	1.0	13	1.2	1.5
51+	M	70	176	2,300[b]	56	1.4	18	1.7	2.0
	F	56	161	1,800[b]	41	1.0	13	1.2	1.5
Pregnant				+300[c]	+20	+0.2	+2	+0.3	+0.5
Lactating				+500	+24	+0.4	+7	+0.6	+0.6

Source:
A Dietary Standard for Canada. Information Canada, Ottawa, 1975. Updated figures may be obtained late 1981 from Health and Welfare Canada, Ottawa K1A 0L2.

[a] Recommendations assume characteristic activity pattern for each age group.

[b] Recommended energy allowance for age 66+ years reduced to 2000 for men and 1500 for women.

[c] Increased energy allowance recommended during second and third trimesters. An increase of 100 kcal per day is recommended during first trimester.

[d] Recommended protein allowance of 2.2 gm/kg body weight for infants age 0-2 mo. and 2.0 gm/kg body weight for those age 3-5 mo. Protein recommendation for infants (0-11 mo.) assumes consumption of breast milk of protein of equivalent quality.

[e] Although recommended intakes are expressed as niacin, it is recognized that approximately 1 mg of niacin is derived from 60 mg of dietary tryptophan.

[f] Recommendations are based on the estimated average daily protein intake of Canadians.

[g] Recommendation given in terms of free folate.

Folate[g]	Vitamin B$_{12}$	Ascorbic Acid	Vitamin A	Vitamin D	Vitamin E$_j$	Calcium	Phosphorus	Magnesium	Iodine	Iron	Zinc
mcg	mcg	mg	mcg RE[i]	mcg$_j$	mg$_j$	mg	mg	mg	mcg	mg	mg
200	3.0	30	1,000	2.5[k]	8	800	800	300	140	10	10
200	3.0	30	800	2.5[k]	6	700	700	250	100	14	9
200	3.0	30	1,000	2.5[k]	8	800	800	300	140	10	10
200	3.0	30	800	2.5[k]	6	700	700	250	100	9	9
+50	+1.0	+20	+100	+2.5[k]	+1	+500	+500	+25	+15	+1[m]	+3
+50	+0.5	+30	+400	+2.5[k]	+2	+500	+500	+75	+25	+1[m]	+7

[h] Considerably higher levels may be prudent for infants during the first week of life to guard against neonatal tryosinemia.

[i] One mcg retinol equivalent (1 mcg RE) corresponds to a biological activity in humans equal to 1 mcg retinol (3.33IU) or 6 mcg β-carotene (10 IU).

[j] One mcg vitamin D is equivalent to 40 IU vitamin D activity. One mg vitamin E is equivalent to 1 mg a-tocopherol.

[k] Most older children and adults receive enough vitamin D from irradiation but 2.5 mcg daily is recommended. This recommended allowance increases 5.0 mcg daily for pregnant and lactating women and for those who are confined indoors or otherwise deprived of sunlight for extended periods.

[l] The intake of breast-fed infants may be less than the recommendation but is considered to be adequate.

[m] A recommended total intake of 15 mg daily during pregnancy and lactation assumes the presence of adequate stores of iron. If stores are suspect of being inadequate, additional iron as a supplement is recommended.

Appendix D—Glossary of Chemicals Commonly Added to Processed Foods

Acacia Gum—see Guar Gum.

Acetic Acid—Vinegar, added to foods to preserve, flavor, or acidify them.

Acetone Peroxide—An aging and bleaching agent used to prepare flour for baking.

Adipic Acid—An acid which is added for a tart flavor to powdered products or drinks.

Agar—A non-digestible, odorless carbohydrate made from seaweed, used as a thickener in ice cream, jam or whipped toppings.

Alginate (Propylene Glycol Alginate)—A thickening or stabilizing agent made from seaweed which is used to maintain the texture of ice cream, cheese, candy, whipped toppings and other non-acidic foods.

Alpha Tocopherol—Vitamin E, added to foods high in fats and oils to keep them from going rancid.

Amino Acetic Acid—see Glycine.

Ammoniated Glycyrrhizin—The flavor component of licorice, also used in root beer or wintergreen flavors. It has been related to high blood pressure and congestive heart failure when eaten in large amounts.

Amylases—Enzymes in cereals that convert starch to sugar. When added to breads or cereals, they develop a sweeter product.

Arabinogalactin (Larch Gum)—A thickener used in many products. It is obtained from the sap of the larch tree.

Artificial Coloring—Most colorings added to foods are made from coal tar dyes, some of which have been shown to be harmful. The presence of an artificial color is usually a good indication of poor quality or low quantity of natural pigments. Few artificial colors, however, are made from natural products.

Artificial Flavoring—Each artificial flavor is a complex mixture of chemicals which is formulated to replace or add to the natural flavor in the food. The presence of artificial flavor usually indicates the absence or near-absence of the food the flavor represents. Examples are artificial orange, vanilla, and banana flavors.

Ascorbic Acid—Vitamin C, added to fruits and their juices to maintain their fresh color and flavor or to add to their nutritional value.

Ascorbyl Palmitate—A fat-soluble chemical form of ascorbic acid, used primarily in high-fat foods as a preservative.

Azodicarbonamide—A maturing agent used in preparing flour before baking.

Benzoate of Soda, Benzoic Acid—see Sodium Benzoate.

Benzolyl Peroxide—An agent which bleaches flour, usually used in conjunction with a maturing agent. Besides destroying the vitamin E in the flour, there are no harmful side effects.

Beta Carotene—a forerunner of vitamin A. It has a yellow color, so can be added as a coloring agent or a nutrition supplement to desserts or imitation dairy products.

Bromelain—see Meat Tenderizers.

Brominated Vegetable Oil—Used mainly in soft drinks to help disperse artificial flavor in water. It is toxic and the amount allowed is therefore restricted. Only heavy consumption of pop might increase its level to the point of danger.

Butylated Hydroxyanisole (BHA) and Butylated Hydroxytoluene (BHT)—These are added to foods containing fats and oils to increase shelf life. Although commonly used in many products, often the necessity of their use is questionable.

Caffeine—A substance which occurs naturally in coffee, tea, cocoa, and kola beans (which are used in making cola drinks). This chemical is a known stimulant and can be habit-forming. Additional amounts may be added to soft drinks over and above that which occurs naturally. Heavy consumption of caffeine-containing foods could lead to addiction to these foods.

Calcium Lactate—see Lactic Acid.

Calcium Phosphates—These are added to a large variety of foods as preservatives or as sources of calcium and phosphorus, both of which are necessary for healthy bones.

Calcium and Sodium Propionate—Chemicals used to prevent the growth of bacteria and mold in baked goods.

Calcium Sorbate—see Sorbic Acid.

Carob Bean Gum—see Locust Bean Gum.

Carrageenan—A stabilizer or thickening agent made from a type of seaweed. This product is often used in commercially prepared milk products, desserts, and until recently ready-to-feed baby formula. There have been some reports linking carrageenan to some forms of cancer.

Casein—The protein from milk. It is added for whiteness and texture to real and artificial dairy products and a variety of food products.

Chewing Gum Base—A product made from natural or synthetic substances, used to give a chewy texture. It has no nutritional value.

Chlorine (Cl_2) and Chlorine Dioxide (ClO_2)—Both are gases which are used to age and bleach flour. There is usually no residue of these gases left after baking.

Citric Acid—It is the substance that gives citrus fruits their acid flavor. It is usually used in citrus or fruit flavored drinks and foods.

Corn Syrup—A sweet syrup used to sweeten or thicken products. It can be dried and used in powdered products, and is then called corn syrup solids. It contains mainly the sugar glucose, which is not as sweet as table sugar, sucrose.

Cysteine—An amino acid (protein component) which occurs naturally in foods. It can be added to foods to prevent oxygen from destroying vitamin C, or to improve the quality of a dough.

Dextrin—A breakdown product of starch which is used to thicken or prevent crystallization in food products.

Dextrose (glucose)—A sugar which does not have all the sweetness of table sugar—see Invert Sugar and Sugar below.

Diethylpyrocarbonate(DEPC)—Prevents the growth of micro-organisms in alcoholic beverages and soft drinks.

Dimethylpolysiloxane (Methyl Silicone, Methyl Polysilicone)—An apparently harmless substance added to many foods to prevent foaming. It is often used in antacid tablets to help absorb extra gas formed in the stomach and intestine due to indigestion.

Dioctylsodium Sulfo-Succinate (DSS)—A chemical added to some powdered products to help them dissolve in water.

Disodium EDTA—see EDTA.

Disodium Guanylate (GMP) and Disodium Inosinate (IMP)—Flavor enhancers added to many prepared foods or mixes. In the same family as monosodium glutamate (MSG).

EDTA (Ethylenediaminetetraacetate or Disodium EDTA)—An apparently harmless substance added to many food products to prevent rancidity in fats and discoloration in fruits and vegetables and to trap any minute particles of metal that may have entered the food during processing.

Ergosterol (Vitamin D)—A natural product in yeast and mold that is converted to vitamin D by ultra violet irradiation. This is the form in which vitamin D is added to milk.

Ethyl Vanillin—see Vanillin.

Ferrous Gluconate—A source of iron that is used in vitamin supplements and fortified foods. It is also used to color black olives.

Ficin—see Meat Tenderizers.

Fumaric Acid—It is added to many foods to give a tart flavor.

Furcelleran—A vegetable gum product which acts as a gelling agent in milk puddings and a thickening agent in other foods.

Gelatin—A natural gelling agent which is made from collagen, an animal protein.

Gluconic Acid—A leavening agent often used in cake mixes and as an acid in powdered gelatin desserts or soft drink mixes.

Glycerine (Glycerol)—Used as a moisturizer, often in candies to prevent them from becoming dried out and hard.

Glycine (Aminoacetic Acid)—An amino acid (part of protein) that can be added to artificially sweetened soft drinks to lessen the bitter after-taste of saccharine.

Guar Gum, Gum Arabic (Acacia Gum, Gum Senegal)—These are vegetable gums which are widely used as thickening agents or stabilizers.

Gum Ghatti—A vegetable gum used as an emulsifier, to keep water and fat layers from separating in products like salad dressing.

Gum Senegal—see Guar Gum.

Hydrogenated Vegetable Oil or Shortening—Oil (or a mixture of oils) that has been hardened by bubbling hydrogen into it. It is a saturated fat. Saturated fat in the diet is associated with high blood cholesterol and risk of heart disease.

Hydrolyzed Vegetable Protein (HVP)—A vegetable protein which has been broken down into amino acids and acts as a flavor enhancer.

Hydroxylated Lecithin—An emulsifier and stabilizer used in baked goods, ice cream and margarine. It is formed by treating lecithin with a peroxide.

Imitation Beef and Chicken Flavors—These are formulations containing hydrolyzed vegetable protein, monosodium glutamate, sugars, vegetable fat, amino acids, disodium inosinate, disodium guanylate (chicken only) and modified starch.

Invert Sugar—(see Sugar Below)—Mixture of glucose and fructose resulting from inversion (or digestion) of table sugar. It is added to foods as a sweetener. Glucose has 70% the sweetening power of sugar, while fructose has 170% of the sweetening power of sugar.

Karaya Gum—Natural vegetable gum from the sterculia tree, used as an emulsifier to prevent fats from separating from water or meat.

Lactic Acid (Calcium Lactate)—The acid is added to foods to keep them acid or to give them a tart flavor. Calcium Lactate inhibits discoloration of fruits and vegetables and improves the properties of dry milk powders and condensed milk.

Lactose—The sugar in milk is used in some products where not much sweetness is desired. It has one-sixth the sweetening power of sugar.

Larch Gum—see Arabinogalactin.

Lecithin—An emulsifier that is added to many fatty foods to prevent separation of fat and water.

Locust Bean Gum (Carob Bean Gum, St. John's Bread)—It is obtained from the bean of the carob tree and is used as a stabilizer in foods to maintain their texture.

Malic Acid—It is used to give a tart flavor to fruits or fruit-flavored products.

Malt Flour—Germinated barley or wheat that has been dried and milled. It contains enzymes that digest starch to the sugars, maltose and glucose. It increases solubility and sweetness in a food.

Mannitol—It is used as a sweetener in diet or low calorie food products.

Meat Tenderizers (Bromelain, Papain, Ficin)—Enzymes from plants which act on meat (mainly the gristle) and begin digesting it, making it more tender.

Methyl Silicone and Methyl Polysilicone—see Dimethylpolysiloxane.

Modified Starch—Starch that has been treated chemically or physically to change its gel strength, color, clarity, or stability. Some treatments do not change the nutritional value of the starch while others affect its digestibility.

Mono and Diglycerides—These are added to many foods containing high levels of fat to help stabilize their texture.

Monosodium Glutamate—A salt of an amino acid often added to foods to give them a more pronounced flavor. Excessive levels are known to cause transient episodes of headaches and flushes in some people.

Niacin (Vitamin B_3)—A vitamin that is necessary for the normal metabolism of carbohydrates, protein and fat.

Oxystearin—A modified fatty acid added to vegetable oils to prevent them from getting cloudy in cold temperatures.

Papain—see Meat Tenderizers.

Pectin—It forms a natural gel in jams and jellies and is often added for this purpose.

Polysorbate 60, 65, 80—Emulsifiers added to many foods to keep the fat and water from separating.

Potassium Bromate—It is added to flour as an aging agent to improve its baking qualities.

Potassium Iodide, Cuprous Iodide, Potassium or Calcium Iodate—Sources of iodine, which are added to table salt. Iodine is a nutrient that is needed in the diet to prevent goiter.

Potassium or Calcium Iodate—These are conditioning agents often added to flour to improve its baking qualities.

Potassium Sorbate—see Sorbic Acid.

Propyl Gallate—It is added to fats and oils, often along with BHT or BHA to prevent rancidity.

Propylene Glycol Alginate—see Alginate.

Propylene Glycol and Fatty Acid Esters—These are added to foods to maintain their moisture and content to carry flavoring substances.

Quillaia—An extract from the soapbark tree used to stabilize the foam in root beer.

Reduced Iron—A source often used in the enrichment of flour and cereals.

Riboflavin (Vitamin B_2)—A B vitamin that is needed for the metabolism of protein.

Saccharin—An artificial sweetener used in low-calorie products. It has a sweetening power of 300-500 times that of sugar but has no caloric value.

Saint John's Bread—see Locust Bean Gum.

Salt (Common salt or table salt)—Added to foods for flavoring effect. Large intakes have been associated with the development of high blood pressure.

Silicone Dixoide—Added to salt and other dry products to keep them dry and to prevent caking.

Sodium Benzoate (Benzoate of Soda, Benzoic Acid)—A preservative used to kill bacteria in acid foods.

Sodium Bisulfite—see Sulfur Dioxide.

Sodium Iron Pyrophosphate—Source of iron which is needed for healthy blood. The availability of iron to the body from sodium iron pyrophosphate is relatively lower than it is from other sources of iron such as ferric sulfate or fine mesh reduced iron. Shortage of adequate sources of iron in the diet leads to anemia.

Sodium Nitrate and Sodium Nitrite—Preservatives added to processed or cured meat products to kill bacteria and to enhance the red color of the meat. Nitrites are known to form nitrosamines which are carcinogenic. Thus, the amounts permitted in food are restricted by law.

Sodium Propionate—see Calcium and Sodium Propionate.

Sodium Sorbate—see Sorbic Acid.

Sorbic Acid (Calcium, Sodium or Potassium Sorbate)—These are added to acid foods to prevent the growth of mold and fungus.

Sorbitan Monostearate—An emulsifier added to dessert products and candies to stabilize their fat.

Sorbitol—A sugar-type sweetener, with almost two-thirds the sweetening power of sugar. Since it is absorbed slowly it is used in foods for diabetics.

Sugar (Sucrose)—Table sugar prepared from sugar cane or sugar beet. It is added to foods as a sweetener. High sugar consumption is associated with obesity, hypertension, diabetes, dental caries, and risk of heart disease.

Sulfur Dioxide, Sodium Bisulfate—Preservatives that prevent discoloration, used mainly in fruit and vegetable products and in wine.

Tannin, Tannic Acid—A chemical mixture found in tea, coffee, and cocoa. It can be added as an ingredient of artificial flavors.

Textured Vegetable Protein (TVP), Isolated Soy Protein—Soy protein products that are in powdered or textured form, often used to replace or blend with ground meat.

Thiamin (Vitamin B_1)—A vitamin that is needed for the normal metabolism of carbohydrate.

Vanillin, Ethyl Vanillin, Vanilla—These are the flavoring extracts made from the beans of the vanilla plant or are synthetic vanillin flavors.

Vitamin A—see Beta Carotene.

Vitamin B_1—see Thiamin.

Vitamin B_2—see Riboflavin.

Vitamin B_3—see Niacin.

Vitamin C—see Ascorbic Acid.

Vitamin D—see Ergosterol.

Vitamin E—see Alpha Tocopherol.

Index